Notes from a Non-Expectant Mother

A Journey to Motherhood through IVF and Adoption

Loretta Lupi-Lawrence

Notes from a Non-Expectant Mother
A Journey to Motherhood through IVF and Adoption

Copyright © *Loretta Lupi-Lawrence,* 2025
All Rights Reserved

This book is subject to the condition that no part of this book is to be reproduced, transmitted in any form or means; electronic or mechanical, stored in a retrieval system, photocopied, recorded, scanned, or otherwise. Any of these actions require the proper written permission of the author.

Disclaimer

Notes from a Non-Expectant Mother

A Journey to Motherhood through IVF and Adoption is an intimate and unflinching memoir that chronicles Loretta Lupi-Lawrence's deeply personal journey through infertility, IVF treatment, miscarriage, and adoption. While the narrative ultimately celebrates resilience, love, and the creation of a family, it explores emotionally challenging themes with raw honesty.

Readers should be aware that this book contains candid discussions of baby loss, including the author's experiences with miscarriage and failed IVF cycles, which may be distressing for those who have undergone similar struggles. Additionally, the memoir addresses themes of trauma, grief, mental health, and the realities of adopting children from abusive backgrounds.

The author's reflections are drawn from lived experience, though some names and identifying details have been altered to protect privacy. This memoir is a testament to the complexities of motherhood, but readers are encouraged to engage with it mindfully, particularly if the subject matter resonates with personal experiences of loss or trauma.

For Our Twins;

Dolly & Buddie you grew in our hearts & we will forever love you unconditionally,

Always

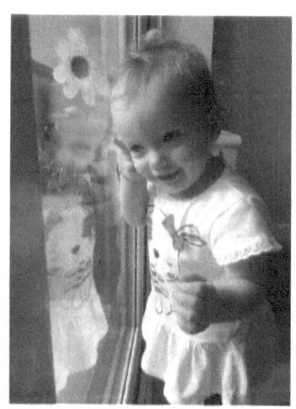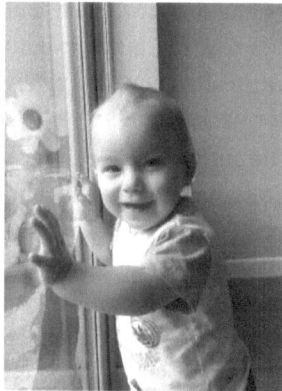

Contents

Disclaimer	3
Foreword	7
The Waiting Game	10
Part One In the Beginning	16
Glory Days	17
The Path Begins	22
Let the Good Times Roll!	29
Family Loading	33
Pregnant Pause	40
Part Two The IVF years	44
In Vitro Fertilisation	45
We Go Again	55
Once More Unto The Breach	60
Pregnant	66
The Bit In Between	67
The Knockout Round	76
The Fog of Grief	85
Therapy, My New Best Friend	90
Injecting Colour Not Meds	94
Part Three The Adoption Years	99
Welcome To Social Services	100
Foster To Adopt	110
Training Begins	117
Save The Worst Until Last	128
The Application Form	138

Lupi By Name, Loopy By Nature	144
The Panel	165
Parties, Catalogues & Resumés	174
The Final Furlong	180
Postscript	187
Acknowledgement	188

Foreword

If you were to ask me what parenting is all about for us, I am likely to ask you to imagine a makeshift dusty road full of potholes, crickets incessantly chirping from dry scrub on the verges. The relentless heat of the midday sun shining in your eyes rendering you blind to see the road ahead. Up ahead there are more than a few hairpin bends to navigate with not a lot of room for manoeuvre when an oncoming vehicle is hurtling towards you. It leaves you feeling completely out of control. I travel this road in a beaten-up old car which incidentally has had just the one fairly careless owner its whole life and a knackered chassis as a result – worth noting that I ordered a brand-new vehicle, but this is what I got. Dramatic? Well yes, that's me, always skirting around the drama despite trying my very best to be a more levelheaded 'normal' person.

It is fair to say that being a mother to twins has aged me beyond measure, both mentally and physically. Too many times to mention, I have had to search inward to find some remnants of strength and often dig even deeper for courage to keep momentum. I have physically aged. I used to beam proudly at the number of times people would say, 'Wow, I thought you were ten years younger!' My brain is now so full of stuff, mostly useless, that I have morphed into an unrecognisable, forgetful, quite scatterbrained, unkempt woman. I can never find my keys and I forget birthdays (actually, that is not really a new thing) coffee dates with friends are frequently missed and I often wonder why our bank account looks sparse when it occurs to me that I have, in fact, forgotten to invoice clients that month.

Long gone are those heady days of thinking only of the immediate and lurching from party to work to long, luxurious lie ins and impromptu trips away - caring not a jot for savings, the future, or consequences. The job title that is motherhood has not remotely been an easy role from the moment the twins burst into our lives. It was a shock to my system suddenly having two active toddlers around. I thought I was prepared for it, but that could not have been further from the truth. I have watched my friends juggling babies and careers with such ease, I have seen the Instagram wonder mothers killing it parenting and looking to die for in their latest gifted PR items. For the first two years, I easily replaced my entire wardrobe for joggers and baggy jumpers, self-care went flying out the window (hairy legs anyone?), I missed my friendships as they steered clear of this new, slightly hysterical person, I replaced work with toilet training, and I grabbed all my energy from chocolate, eating my feelings as I felt completely out of my depth. At one point, I definitely thought I was going insane from lack of sleep and desperately trying to figure out how to attach to my children, all the while constantly thinking, why did the social workers entrust me with this job?

Despite all of this, somehow motherhood has become easily the most rewarding job I have ever had. I must admit, now that I am six years in, I really am a better person for having them in my life but, in truth, I am only just finding solid ground beneath my feet. As I went through the stages of writing this memoir, I found that despite it all I would not swap my motherhood journey for any other nor for the moon on a stick.

Becoming a mother is the biggest honour I can think of, and I am very aware that sounds like yet another classic cliché that is kicked around on social media at the mere mention of the word parenting. As I watch my children grow and explore, it feels like the most wonderful privilege of all, teaching them all you know, passing on a lifetime of experiences and traditions for them to pocket and use when they need them. Banking every experience in your mind, tucking it away somewhere special to pull out when a pick me up is needed, as if it is a piece of priceless treasure.

Most mothers I would imagine feel and connect with this joy; most mothers also talk about the struggle of parenting being 'real' but how motherhood is the best job in the world. I am not alone in this. I wonder how many mothers feel like a knackered old car most days and whether their route to children was as full of potholes as mine was.

I am not most mothers; we do not have a similar story; our journey is not like any other journey. Motherhood is not just my story, it is *our* story. The story of how I came to be a mother and how the twins found a mother were endured by moments of chaos, confusion, relentless pain, and sadness. Of violent and abusive episodes. Of grief and trauma. And ultimately, an unconditional love that can withstand and protect them from any more storms.

I am Loretta, a mother to two incredible souls who not only need me to love them but alongside parenting to untangle the fibres of life that happened before I met them. To understand and share their pain, to work it all out with them, to protect them from any more harm and to stop the terror in their nightmares. The word 'victim' speaks so loudly; however, in truth, that is what they are. Our twins are victims of adults who should have known better. We cannot take that from them or bear the pain for them, only ease the severity of scars that are ingrained in every cell in their body and teach them that they can rise up and look forward to a beautiful, safe life.

This is our story. How we became bound together forever through endurance, humour, and, above all, love.

The Waiting Game

Scanning my emails, as I munched my way through another unsatisfyingly boring salad at lunchtime, I was looking for one email in particular. Again. I had become obsessive about this one email arriving. I did not really expect there to be one waiting for me today, but I lived in eternal hope. I was continuously being told to be patient by everyone around me, 'when the time is right, it will come.' *Time. How much more time was I meant to wait?*

Except inside this lunch break, there it was, sat snugly between an email from British Gas containing an energy statement and an Amazon Echo Dot recommendation. Louisa's emails stood out to me as if they had flashing lights on them. I just stared at it, blinking at me, fork midway to my mouth, as I registered the enormity of what waited inside this email for us. I had waited so long for this email but now I couldn't open it; I just continued to stare at it until the words blurred. Slowly, my brain unfroze itself, salad easily abandoned; I clicked on the email to open it, noticing instantly an attachment. I dismissed the niceties of the greeting and scanned the email for the information I needed. There in black and white stood thirteen words that I knew in my core would change the course of our lives forever. '**There are children, twins actually, that I think are suited to you both.** I have attached a photo and a basic biography. Let me know if you wish to proceed.' I am pretty sure my heart and my breath stopped whilst the picture downloaded from the email. Nothing existed around me other than the screen and a pounding in my ears; it had all fallen away. It must have only taken seconds to download, but it is fair to say I am impatient, even at the best of times. *Why is our internet connection so bloody slow?* My screen finally filled with two beautiful smiling toddlers playing at a patio window. Both stood up, small palms flat on the window for stability, having just learnt to walk. A cheeky grin on one and a big smile on the other as they looked at something beyond the pane of glass. Boy and girl twins. My stomach lurched and tears stung the back of my eyes and right there in that moment, I was certain of two things. The first, these were our children; I felt it with every fibre of my body. The second thing unfolding in my brain was that they are the 'why'. These two beautiful, innocent souls are why our IVF attempts failed. I understood our happy fate as if the final piece of our puzzle had finally been located and clicked into place. I sobbed and laughed at the same time with relief, possibly looking like some kind of unhinged mad woman.

Was it possible to feel unconditional love from a photo on a screen? Apparently, yes.

Rereading the email in full this time, I quickly learnt from the rest of the email that the twins had three older siblings and a younger one too. They had been taken away at eleven months old from abusive parents and were now under the care of a fosterer. The twins were now fourteen months old and were just learning to walk. That was it; that was all I knew. I read it again, and again until I knew it by heart.

I was in the back room of our shop; I watched Henri cutting his client's hair from the doorway. My body was jittery, transferring weight from foot to foot, a mascara-streaked, tear-stained face, the memory of the photograph held in my mind's eye, I was visibly shaking. *What a mess. Pull it together for goodness' sake, people are starting to furrow their brows at you.* He was nearly done with the cut. He turned. He beamed at me and then, just for a small beat, his gaze lingered on my frame. I saw his face register; he knew what I knew. He grinned and finished his client with less pomp than normal. We did it. We have children I blurted out as soon as he reached the doorway.

"Children? What do you mean?"

"Yup," I am beaming, "I am not joking, it's twins!"

I led him to the screen that still held the picture of the twins grinning from it. I could feel his heart swelling from the intense squeeze of my hand in his; he had become a little giddy too.

"Both of them? We are going to have both?" I filled in the gaps from what little I knew and together we phoned Louisa to say yes. *Buzzkill, of course it is an answer machine.* I eye rolled and we left a message, followed by an emailed reply too, and until Henri stopped me, I would have phoned again, and again until she picked up, proving that I had learnt nothing about being patient.

Naively, I expected the next part of the process to be plain sailing, as if nothing about our journey had taught me anything at all. Louisa finally called us back, explaining that there were two other couples looking to adopt the twins as well as us, and we had to enter what can only be described as a bidding war. Not with money but with ourselves and our lifestyles. Never has it been more important to be able to offer the best. Louisa was our bidder against two other bidding social workers. They had to hold a meeting to hash it out in a room with a lead social worker at the helm overseeing the discussion. We had to wait a week for it to be organised and held. A whole seven days. One hundred and sixty-eight hours.

I didn't sleep. How could I sleep? I kept looking at the photos of these children - not that I needed to, as I knew every inch of their faces already. The older twin, the girl, her grin at something making her smile outside, one tiny hand by her head, her pudgy finger pointing, the tuft of soft, golden hair curling upwards on her head and a rogue curl sticking out behind her ear. Sea blue eyes, amused. A cute tiny button nose between her rosy, red cheeks. The boy, resting his hand on the patio window, looking at the same something outside, his dark brown almond-shaped eyes glistened, giving away his joy. His blonde hair, thin and wispy, had created a little mound on the top of his head. Innocent faces that had already been through too much pain.

I was frustrated and, not for the first time, feeling utterly useless. Not only could I not have a hand in fighting for them to come home with us, but now I was feeling insecure, scared and a little bit angry at being introduced to children that we could potentially lose out on to another couple who were probably feeling as wretched as I do right now. *Do the other couples feel this way too? Four people are going to have their hearts crushed, will have to start their search again. Please, please don't let it be us.*

Before the week was up, four days in, we had a phone call from Louisa. The twins had a tiny four week old baby sibling also up for adoption. Louisa questioned whether we would want to go for her as well, to maybe keep the three siblings together, although there was no guarantee. No question. Of course, we would. Louisa sent over her file. A tiny, innocent, beautiful little baby. Wrapping our heads around potentially two children was mind-blowing, but three? A day later Louisa called to say it had been decided that their small sibling would be allocated to a different couple. Our flat was not quite laid out as the adoption rules dictated it to be, with one bedroom being upstairs. The requirement is that all bedrooms should be on one level and next to each other. Strangely, though, it didn't feel like another disappointment to digest. In all honesty, we were not sure we would cope with three children under two; it was the right decision. We knew it then, and we definitely know it now; the twins' youngest sibling is living in a joy filled world with so much love given by her own wonderful adoptive parents.

The days slowly rolled on. No call came. I carried my phone in my hand, ready to hear our fate, hour after hour. My internal monologue was in turmoil as I lurched from the negative thoughts that ranged from perhaps losing the twins to the bubbling anger at the process. *How much more can we take; I think I need someone to put me out of my misery before I self-combust. I should be calmer; let's meditate and breathe this frustration out. Where's my yoga mat? I'll just do it on the sofa. Ok. Clear your mind. What if we lose them? Ahhh, they are not ours anyway. Stop! Shh! I blame myself; I got us here in the first place; maybe if you had eaten a better diet. Shh! Concentrate. Think of nothing. Is that my phone ringing? Where is my phone? This is not going to work.* I actively shoved down old thoughts, blaming myself for not having got us here sooner in the first place and went for a run.

Wednesday morning and the sky heavy with expected rain, I was emerging from the bank having completed a mundane admin job for our shop; my mind momentarily occupied compiling a shopping list of food we needed later as I crossed the road. My phone started ringing. Typically, after days of having that phone burning a hole in my hand, it was now buried at the bottom of my shoulder tote. I threw the bag on the pavement and dived in. I missed the call. Louisa. *Damn it!* I called back as quickly as my fingers could unlock the phone. There, on the street, wrapped against the cold of the November day, sandwiched between the ordinary, the bank, and a bookshop, I received life-changing news. Everyone and everything around me blurred, my eyes suddenly full of tears. The twins, if we were still sure we wanted them, were now our children. A family had been birthed at that moment in time under the grey sky on the pavement of the high street.

What a picture I must have been had you not known me and our story. A woman wrapped in a woolly scarf and a bright orange winter coat, an open tote at her feet with a few escaped parts of her life scattered beside it, a bunch of keys, a banking book, a mini pack of tissues, some loose mints, and a clattering steel water bottle as it rolled away from her. Tears cascading down her face, leaving dark and smudged black mascara on her cheeks. A smile as wide as it could stretch. Twirling in circles, dancing around her now abandoned tote and repeating words of gratitude to the caller on the end of the phone she had to her ear.

I picked up the items I had thrown out of my tote, threw them back in, not caring for the items, and ran. I ran up the high street to our shop. I paused at the door as I gathered the information I needed to impart and burst into the shop pulling Henri to the back room. Breathing hard from the uphill run. "We did it. We did it. We are parents. The twins are coming home." *Wait. What? Wow, we are going to be parents.* Not parents that birthed their children but parents that fought hard for years. Parents that stood strong from the path they had taken. Parents born from a journey that turned them inside out. In that moment we felt the relief course through us. We clung to each other, our hearts beating hard and fast whilst we digested the news; the babies from the photograph that we had fallen hopelessly in love with were coming home.

Part One
In the Beginning

Glory Days

I remember being a kid so vividly; for my younger sister and I, it was a glorious existence; we were lucky enough to enjoy carefree days of long, hot summer holidays, running through sprinklers shrieking with delight; birthdays and Christmas were momentous occasions, arguing and playing in equal measure with each other; trips to the South of France and Northern Italy's Riveria, finding adventure in everything; navigating private school with new friends. Dreaming big was my thing. My relatives used to say if I did not have my head in a book, it was in the clouds creating exciting adventures for when I was a grown up.

Childhood life was good. I had very loving, hard-working parents and my grandparents lived in the annexe attached to our house too. My whole world under one roof. Our house was my father's vision, which he built from his mind on the architect's table. The house, as beautiful as it was inside, was not what I loved the most. It was the garden. I loved being outside, whether it was autumn, and I was playing in the leaves; or winter and building a mountain of snowballs; or Summer helping out with the vegetable plot.

Our back garden began from the steps down from the large, raised patio where we ate barbecues in the summer evenings and played 'Benny', our family card game; a vast front lawn with uniformed lines mowed into the lush soft green grass, old fruit trees lining the edges to block out the ugly boundary fence that sat behind it. The deep borders at the far end against the wall that adjoined next door's garden, where an abundance of flowering plants spilt colour onto the lawn, plenty of room for playing, make-believe and hiding amongst the trees and taller shrubs. Around to the side and along the ancient crumbling wall, the garden narrowed slightly before flushing out again to where the log and coal house sat - always fully stocked to fuel the fireplaces. The vegetable patch behind that, which could be viewed from the kitchen window, lay raised and butted up right next to our neighbours the other side of the old wall who were laid to rest in their well-tended graves in the churchyard. The garden then led round to the front. To the left was a gravelled small lane where, at the end of it, Papa had built a smaller cottage for guests. This building sat at the top end with a view of our fields in front of it. The fields were rented out to our local farmer for rearing his lambs in spring; every season, we were invited to bottle-feed them. The joy of when the daffodils and bluebells started to pop their colours in the garden brought about excitement as we knew the lambs were soon arriving. We loved hand-feeding them milk, the lambs sucked and pulled hungrily at the bottles we held with two hands, we laughed as they nearly pulled us over in their quest to satisfy their hunger.

Moving away from the cottage there was a small lawn in front of the patio window that my grandparents looked out onto. Two enormous plane trees stood proudly on the edge of that lawn, I used to lay between them in those long summer days immersed in a book, often looking up at them, marvelling at how they still stood so tall and proud after a warplane had crashed between them in the Second World War. I often think of them now, drawing on what they stood for; strength and resilience.

Just beyond those trees, we were privileged enough to have a tennis court that sat at the bottom of one of our fields. I remember feeling frustrated as no one would play tennis with me, so Papa built me a wall in one half of the court to hit the ball against to stop me from incessantly asking him to scrap the court and put a pool in instead. Angela, my younger sister, used to rollerblade around and around the smooth tarmac, perfecting her rolling stride one summer; a standout memory as I watched on with pride as she got faster and more skilled, although I often wondered who she was competing against. A stone's throw from the gate to the tennis court stood a beautiful gazebo, not the pop-up kind you see at markets but one with pillars made from old red bricks and a slated roof that displayed beautiful and fragrant white creeping wisteria in bloom. We used to leave homemade lemonade in jugs in the shade there, ready to quench our thirst after playing on the court.

The driveway's biggest feature was the horse chestnut tree spreading its branches wide like an opened umbrella in the centre of the lawned roundabout on the driveway; in the autumn, this tree boasted its health and rewarded us with hundreds of conkers to play with and for my mother to collect and line along windowsills inside the house like round shiny soldiers ready to see off any unwelcome spiders seeking winter warmth. The driveway led down the slope to the double garage doors, where in the early learning-to-skate days, Angela once broke her out-of-control rolling with her nose. It was accessed via the long track leading from the hotel my parents owned. Right beside the driveway gate warning people to 'Beware of the Dog' was an old weeping willow tree we used to hide under when we waited for guests to arrive, bursting out our hellos when they emerged from their cars.

Yeah, we really did have the most incredibly diverse playground and safe home to play out our childhood days. We did not know how lucky we were to come home from school to our gated house full of love and everything we ever needed. There wasn't another world away from this one, was there? One of the games that I would role-play as a child was that of mummies and babies with my dolls. I was the mummy obviously and my children, aka my doll and my number one confidante teddy whose fur was loved hard to thin and patchy, and a boy doll called Celestino borrowed from my sister, would be born into the same house set up as my own, except with the addition of a pool and swing and slide set. Hours upon hours, I would make believe how my future children's lives would play out; there would be three children, two girls, and a boy, all happy and safe with all they needed. They would grow and conquer the world on the stage or fly cabin crew to exotic locations. Those days when I daydreamed about becoming a mother, it was so whimsical, so naïve, so fairytale. My childhood daydream eventually became a reality, a mother to twins, a boy, and a girl, but that similarity is where it ends. As a child I would have recoiled in horror at what came with this future chapter of my life. Not in my wildest nightmares would my make-believe children have seen and experienced what our twins have.

My childhood home stands in stark contrast to what the twins were born into and endured, that is, until the social workers finally came with the police, raided the flat and took all of them to safety.

....

Jane and Andrew brought the twins home from the hospital eight days after they were born to a two-bedroomed, top-floor flat given to them by the council.

Their village is picturesque and sits amongst the rolling hills of the English countryside. A busy and noisy but small estate at the top of a steep hill whose street, before the flats loom into view, is lined with decent-sized red brick houses with front and back gardens, including a little space for each car per household on a petite driveway. For the flats at the top of the hill, they were not greeted by a red brick driveway but the bin area for their block, where a lengthy list of dos and don'ts written by the local housing association is hammered to the wooded fence that contained them. These rules will greet any tenant or visitor before finding the pathway to the entrance running alongside it. Sometimes, in the summer months, the smell of rotting food can be eye-watering before they are emptied. Before finding the entrance to the flats, there is a small communal untended area of patchy grass, the mud visible, where three tired, shared washing lines stand on the left and on the right weaves the weedy, uneven path to the communal door entrance. Out-of-control brambles and invasive bindweed mark off the area given to the families that live there. There are some discarded and faded plastic toys scattered in the grass that you can imagine the younger tenants playing with as the parent sought out a space on the washing line to hang laundry. Litter is strewn on the ground as the bins lose their grip on some of the rubbish stashed inside them.

Inside their flat, it was dark and unclean, with clutter and mess covering every surface. The living room hosted a blue two-seater sofa clashing with stained cream wallpaper with its gigantic pattern of repeated burgundy flowers. The hub in the room was the television, where all their gadgets and connecting cords were strewn around it, ready to be plugged in on a whim at a moment's notice. Surfaces were filled with keys, rubbish, fresh and dirty nappies, used dishes, cigarettes, scattered tobacco bits and thick dust; the remnants of their life. Noticeably missing were toys or books from three older siblings already living out their childhood inside those walls. Two bedrooms and now five children. Jane and Andrew had no income and relied on benefits to live on, to feed not only their children but their addictions too. Life was indeed tough, and unbeknownst to them they were already on the social services radar.

The Path Begins

I met Henri two years after I chose Wiltshire as a place to base myself after years of living in London. It was near my small childhood hometown but there was some distance; I wasn't quite ready to be living back there again, it still felt claustrophobic. I felt like I had failed in chasing down a satisfying, long-lasting career, I was not ready to admit it to my family, so I lived as close to them as I felt comfortable with. I will never really know why I chose this city as a place to live in, I had so many other options open to me, I simply had a sense it would be the right place to be in. The only time I had ever visited this city before was as a child to buy my school uniform as the official school uniform shop was based there, and this was long before the internet existed for the ease of online purchasing.

I knew no one in this cathedral city except one old school acquaintance that readily and kindly shared her house with me for around six months until her nightly drinking habit and abusive game-playing boyfriend became too much to bear witness to. At that time in my life, I was carrying around a whole suitcase of trauma that I had chosen to ignore and not deal with, pushing it firmly away whenever it felt close to bursting open, and her initial kindness turned into behaviour that felt really triggering. The years in London had taken a toll on my mental health but at this point, I still continued to think I was just always on the wrong side of luck, that kind of martyrdom suited my head space despite no one being around to listen to it.

Despite that I chose well, such a pretty city steeped in history, with all its twelfth-century original architecture and beautifully manicured parks and public spaces. Plus it never felt like a city after living amongst the chaos of London; boasting an abundance of green space and with just a five-minute drive outside the boundaries lands you deep in rich, hilly, and bountiful Wiltshire countryside.

I yearned to live in one of the city's nearby chocolate box villages, and I even found a little cottage to buy, but I put myself off with the fear that with only my grumpy cat Chloe for company, I would just become an equally grumpy, unapproachable spinster, so instead I plumped for an end of terrace 1940s house on one of the main routes into the centre. Quite the opposite to a chocolate box. My hope was to get a lodger to help alleviate my growing sense of isolation and loneliness. This three up, two down was a place I could call my own (*cliché, I know I seem to be a walking cliché these days*), a haven where I could have somewhere that was mine again.

I had landed a job working in marketing for a finance firm. Everyone who knew me well was baffled by this choice as it was quite possibly the worst job I could have secured as:

a) numbers and money are most definitely not my thing; you only have to look at my GCSE Maths result (or lack of) or my unhealthy-looking bank account and spending habits for that insider information.

b) I despise anything to do with a traditional office, almost like I'm allergic to the environment; the suits, the rules, tethered to a desk, those water cooler moments. No thank you.

c) I had never done any marketing before in my life let alone in finance, an area that frankly could be talking to me in Chinese.

It was, though, the only job I could get.

This was the true definition of 'winging it'. I wasn't actually winging it, of course, as I managed to get fired within four months, surprised I lasted that long, to be honest with you. It may have been the long private meetings I had where, in truth, there was no work done, just moaning about life with my only office ally. It may have been the clash with my younger boss, but overall, it was honestly a huge relief; waiting to be rumbled is nerve-wracking and understated.

My career had been a varied one so far as I bumbled along trying to work out what I wanted to do with my life. Chronologically, there was a low moment of toy demonstrating in the window of Hamleys on Bond Street, a lot of working in different pubs in Soho, call centres in Richmond, nightclub promotions in central London, a fairly decent role at the House of Commons, then after completing my degree in Digital Media and Radio, a producer for a music station, and lastly being part of the advertising team at BBC Worldwide for their toy magazine department before I gave up on the bright lights *(more blinding lights)* of London.

There was also a huge phase of setting up on my own with varying degrees of success. I set up a website building company, Frog Design Ltd and that got me through university financially, quite clever of me even if I say so myself; the work my clients were paying me for simultaneously hitting the assignments required for the course. Then there was Lupilicious (a clever play on my surname at the time but I can't take the credit from my friend Rob, who thought that up on a night out in the pub). It was a bespoke home service offering cleaners, housekeepers, chefs, nannies, dog walkers, and personal assistants, it saw me grow rapidly. However, it became a beast, too big, too quickly for me to handle it. Having to manage an eighteen-strong team of self-employed staff and often demanding and tricky clients was not the life for me, I did, though, manage a good three years with it. Next, I qualified as a life coach, something I was good at but never really took off, my heart was not in it. Alongside all this, I had always written, both for myself and for clients, and of course, I had journaled most of my life. Then, finally, we arrive in the here and now at the grand old age of forty-eight I am not sure how, but I have finally found the confidence to out myself as a writer.

Wind the years back to when I was living in Wiltshire, and after the disastrous job in finance, I applied for a job doing telephone marketing at a media company, calling the last job I was sacked from (and no, I didn't mention that bit!) as 'experience' in marketing. Surely, this would be an easy, mundane job to get me through the funk I was feeling. It was just that. The team was small and friendly, working from an orchard barn, I was ironically surrounded by writers. My new media company employer produced some beautiful national magazines. I remember feeling something like belonging, although that creeping insecurity of how long it would be before I self-sabotage this job started to climb into my psyche before long. There was a good chance that this time, I might not make a mess of it and for now, that suitcase of trauma was still kept firmly shut. A few months in, I was given an opportunity to write an article for one of their magazines and I grabbed the opportunity. I loved it, the research, the interview with the subject and the writing. My article was published, and I felt so hugely proud of myself, but, isn't there always a *but*, I never got offered to write again, so my confidence took a fresh nose dive and I became bored of calling people to see if they wanted to advertise in a directory so I left the little barn of safety that was surrounded by orchards of pretty apple trees to pursue something more familiar, toxic but familiar. Radio.

....

During those years in London, at twenty-six years old, I graduated with a Digital Media and Radio degree from Thames Valley University, which was based in Ealing, west London. I loved all of radio, writing for it, broadcasting, producing others, and creating great content. I was part of the student radio station; it was a buzz. Coming out of university, I walked straight into a small radio station that was in the throes of getting ready for a re-launch and it was here that my suitcase of trauma really started to fill up. The suitcase already contained some darkness from my late childhood, school, friendships gone bad and the like, but this fresh layer that I seemingly invited in contributed heavily to the appearance of the monkey in my head and the rip-roaring anxiety in my chest.

The radio industry in the nineties was a competitive place to be. Everybody wanted to work in this industry; there had been an explosion in the number of stations setting up to broadcast, largely triggered by the introduction of DAB (Digital Audio Broadcasting) in 1995. For those of us graduating at this time, the fight to be seen and employed was brutally competitive. So, I was lucky to walk into a job in a sense; I was so grateful for the security of that job that I was blindsided by what this job held for me. First of all, I was earning a paltry £7,000 a year. I swallowed this salary as I was told that amount is where you start. It's the same everywhere; you need to work your way up the pay ladder. I remember being actually grateful for even being paid at all. The bullying in the workplace started subtly before ramping up, it started by being called to work six days a week, 9 am to sometimes 10 pm. It was exhausting. My job role seemed to have no boundaries; I would be calling record labels, to cleaning loos, to being trained on the scheduling overnight system, to hosting celebrities, producing shows, and fetching the boss's lunch, dinner, or dry cleaning, running his errands, even cleaning his shoes. The boss (we were made to call him 'boss' not by his actual name) was never in a pleasant mood with his staff, only the celebrities, his wife, and the endless stream of girlfriends he brought in. He frequently stubbed his cigarettes out on my freshly printed scripts, flicked ash wherever he walked, yelled in my face, his spittle covering me, his breath stinking of a rancid mix of coffee and alcohol despite his insistence he had been sober for three years. He allowed his celebrity pals to order us around and did cocaine with them in his corner office, whilst playing loud rock 'n roll.

My nerves went first; I was terrified of being shouted at and equally terrified of not doing a good job. I was jittery and on edge from the moment I walked inside the radio building. I often reminded myself of a poorly kept but loyal puppy. We were wowed by the life the industry gave us; I was so caught up in celebrity and its status until it became really obvious that it wasn't all that glamorous. Work parties were plentiful and all of us on the bottom rung of the pay ladder found solace in the free bars.

One summer my parents had travelled up for my Graduation Ceremony and the boss decided I wouldn't be allowed to attend. The more I begged, the more he laughed and said no. A moment of clarity showed me I was not, in fact, in shackles, and I walked out, a slither of courage. I did go back the next day. It took me vomiting from too much free alcohol on the floor of a dirty club bathroom in Camden and two years to leave all that abuse behind. Except I had not left it behind just stuffed the shame and fear into my suitcase.

After that, I may have left that radio building, but I still allowed men in charge to bully me in my work environments, I was still seeking approval, desperately trying to make myself fit in. This awful need in me took me to work with men that could easily dominate me; shocking and terrible things would happen, and I always blamed myself. The self-loathing continued, stuffing itself inside my suitcase. One manager flew into a rage when he noticed me twirling my hair around my finger—a harmless habit I do while thinking. His sudden fury seemed to come out of nowhere, his face turning bright red and his eyes bulging with anger. I swallowed the lump in my throat, blinked back tears in my eyes. The next day, I handed in my notice. Then there was the vile well-known ex-daytime celebrity, took me back to his place on the pretense of talking jobs (*so, so bloody naïve*) only I fell asleep on his sofa and woke in the morning to him climbing on top of me, my clothes in a heap on the floor. I told myself I probably deserved it. Another time, a male client of mine was high on drugs and, having been provoked by a cheating girlfriend, threatened me with a gun. I fled from his premises and once outside on the pavement, the brightness of the day in front of me seemed to strip me bare. The bubble inside me rising up in my chest, the contents of my suitcase threatening to spill out at my feet. Once I was home, I sat on my sofa until the cloak of darkness wrapped itself around me, it occurred to me that I had no one to turn to, no one willing to listen. As I climbed the stairs for bed that night; as I reached the top, a gasp escaped from my throat, my legs crumpled, falling onto the landing carpet, spilling tears down my face, shouting words tumbling out to no one. I found myself calling for my grandfather, who had died five years earlier, I hadn't grieved that loss, I hadn't been able to accept he was gone. The one man in my life that understood me, believed in me. He would squeeze me so tight in his bear hugs anytime I needed them. Those hugs that kept me safe, those hugs that told me I was loved. His thick, calming Yorkshire accent telling me it would all be alright in the end. Would it be alright? Would it really? I sobbed myself to sleep there that night. When I woke stiff and cold, I knew something inside me had snapped, the suitcase was open. I was done. Done. My life could not, and would not, turn out this way. This was not going to be my story.

Let the Good Times Roll!

Radio, as much as I loved presenting it, the sales job I had was a tough place to exist with a tendency for high anxiety and a competitive spirit. I exhausted myself, chasing the numbers. So, I handed my notice in and looked for something else to do. Those last few months working out my notice were tough, I had completely disengaged, struggled to keep my hand in the game and meet any targets or work commitments at all. The night that I had broken apart, I had made my mind up that never again would anyone use me as a puppet or bully me for shits and giggles; I had meant it. I needed to take control and take myself out of an environment that promised to do all that.

Being on my own and finding out who I was at my core was how I wanted to shift my life forward, I was going to be fine, more than fine; in fact, I was going to live my life on my own terms as long as I did not allow myself to be controlled again. I needed to find my voice and to learn to trust myself and not rely on anyone else or fit in specific friendship nooks just because I was lonely. Just the thought of living this way started to make me feel mildly stronger and free. I shed a lot in those last months in radio; controlling male figures, toxic friendships, and the fake version of me, the crowd pleaser, the approval seeker.

....

For the first time in years, I was coming back to the girl who grew up in the countryside, the family orientated daughter, the solid friend. I rediscovered my love of walking in nature, yoga, running, and reading. I started a fresh journal, each word healing me of what came before. I started living. *Have I ever really lived, I mean really felt the intention in my footsteps, made decisions on my own, uninfluenced by anyone else or any part of earlier experience? I want to feel life without drama and trauma; I want to heal and have a simple life. I don't need anyone but me, right? Who am I becoming?*

I had found another job, just a low-key admin-type executive position, filled my spare room with a paying housemate, started going to the gym, and learnt how to protect myself with a course in martial arts.

One warm summer evening my new housemate and I decided at the last minute we would venture into town, taking up the invitation I had had from a vaguely fun guy I had met in a club the week before. He had invited me to a pub in the centre of town to meet his group of friends, listen to some live music, and have a few drinks by the river.

We walked just inside the noisy, packed bar, stopping to scan the room to see if I could see this guy, which was tough as I was not entirely sure what he looked like. *I mean, come on, clubs are dingy, the lighting is shocking and, to be fair, I was tipsy and sweaty from dancing. Okay, he has black-ish hair, average height, stocky. Not really narrowing it down, there are loads of blokes in here that look like that!* It was so crowded that it took me a few minutes before I saw him propping up the bar and chatting up a group of attentive women. I went to move towards him when, at the same time, in another part of the pub, a very tall, handsome, blonde-haired guy grabbed my attention. *Who is that? Oh he is gorgeous. Probably hitched and happy, but he is striking. Oh God, I am staring!* I could not move my eyes past him, the breath in my lungs caught in my throat as he turned to look in my direction and returned my stare. He smiled, I smiled, and we both walked towards the bar. I do not believe in coincidences, so let's call it fate that he turned out to be the club guy's best friend, Henri. He was, in fact, single. That was it. A moment in time that changed both our lives. Years of searching for someone to love and for that to be reciprocated ended in a smattering of seconds inside a poorly lit, crowded pub with a sticky floor from spilt pints and shots of slippery nipples or Jagerbombs, a strong smell of body odour and tinny music so loud conversation was almost ruled out. Who said romance was dead?

On our first date, I noted that everything about him was different from the type of guy I am normally attracted to; he was kind, smiled at me, kept eye contact, was relaxed, funny, chatty, interested in me, and honest. I fell in love with him the moment I saw him in that bar, but the following few dates cemented it for me. I cringe at yet another cliché in my life, but our eyes did meet across a crowded room, how Mills & Boon (pass the bucket). It still makes us laugh at how corny that is and if I had known meeting your soulmate was a simple chance, meeting my younger self could have lived a more anxiety-free existence. We live and learn. *Another cliché.*

Henri was like no one I had dated before or even hung out with; maybe this is why I fell so hard for him. He had been brought up to be a gentleman with morals that he upheld as best he could. He inherited his father's sense of humour, his hardworking ethic, and his ability to connect on a deeper level; from his mother, he had learnt how to nurture and exercise patience – something I definitely do not possess. He has a kindhearted sister, although I hear the early years between them were full of sibling rivalries. Aren't all siblings the same?! He is a barber with a solid reputation. Unlike all the men that had come into my life, arrogant, pushy, controlling, demanding, and selfish, Henri was the exact opposite and thank God for that!

In a nutshell, we had two dates where we just ate and talked, a third meeting his parents on a whim (I was sweaty from a 5km Race for Life run; I make the best impressions,) and on the fourth, he stayed over and never left. After two weeks, we flew to Turkey on holiday for a fortnight. After three months, Digby, our golden retriever puppy, came home to live with us and within the year, we had bought our own house in the countryside. A picturesque whitewashed 1850s three-bedroomed house with a huge garden and an orchard.

Life was happy, fun, and full to the brim with love and laughter. We fully committed to each other and Digby of course, a solid threesome.

Henri opened his own barbershop business at the same time I started my own business, both businesses grew so rapidly we could barely keep up. Three years from when we met, we were married and already two years into trying for a family. It took eight long, hard years of fighting for our family to be born.

Family Loading

Our relationship was always fast-tracked, we met, fell for each other, knew together we stood stronger, and we loved each other in a way that was precious yet unbreakable. We both felt it. We moved fast. *Why wait?* Within those first six months, we talked about having children on and off, how many we would like, genders, and names, concluding that we were in our early thirties, so we should perhaps just start trying. No pressure, just no contraception. We talked about having a big family, three or four children, we talked about adoption combined with having our own little ones, maybe fostering too in the future.

Eighteen months in and still no sign of a pregnancy, nor had we pressed buttons on the adoption process or enquired about fostering, we were content just being together.

One blustery autumnal day, leaves swirling around my feet and my skirt threatening to expose my best underwear that I had worn for a regular smear test appointment. I walked up the deep stone steps and through a big black door not unlike the Number 10 Downing Street door. *Such a grand ornate building feels like the wrong setting for a GP clinic. However, my vagina might appreciate the grandiose.* I snigger at my thoughts as I approach the reception desk. I am sent upstairs to wait for the nurse.

Whilst making small talk (is there any other kind of chat you can hold with your legs open and cold metal spectrum inserted in your vagina?) with the nurse, I mentioned in passing we'd been trying for children for a while with no luck so far.

She frowned, "Are you worried about it? I mean, given your age, are you worried there may be a problem?" I was in my mid-thirties, and it had not occurred to me I should be; my age and my fertility status were not on my radar. I winced as the cold, hard, metal speculum was pushed as far as it could up inside my vagina to reveal my cervix. She turns to grab a small soft brush to take the sample of cells.

"Oh, do you think I should be? I mean, what kind of thing should I be worried about?" I had moved up onto my elbows now. She gently pushed me back down to lying so she could get a better view.

"I'll make an appointment for you with the doctor, see if we can get the ball rolling, it can't hurt to put your mind at rest and make sure it's all working." She laughed uncomfortably and pulled out the speculum that made an even more uncomfortable sucking noise. "All done for another year." She snapped off her latex gloves and started to wash her hands. My annual duty to my vagina is complete.

Put my mind at rest. What does that mean? That morning, the nurse triggered a new alarm in my head and my old demon, anxiety, started to creep its thick black smoke in at the corners of my life once more. A small fire had started in my brain. That familiar feeling of dread started to curl its way back into my life. This time I was not being controlled by the arrogant, the self-important, the overpowering in my life, but my own body felt like it could be turning against me.

From that day and still no sign of pregnancy, I always had a sense it was me, my fault, of course, it was *my* body that had failed us. Confirmation after initial tests were done found that it was, in fact, likely to be me. Not one of the professionals I saw could ever give me a real tangible explanation as to why, just a bunch of guessing possibilities, I needed more tests.

Since I started menstruating as an early teenager, I have suffered from extremely painful periods, the kind that takes your breath away and make you double over. As a thirteen-year-old, I was prescribed enormous tablets that I crushed up and put between two slices of bread, slathered in condensed milk to mask the taste in order to swallow them. My mother used to call them the horse tablets. Then, at age fourteen, I was put on a contraceptive pill in a bid to minimise the pain. Neither the painkiller nor the contraceptive pill worked, but despite that, I was instructed to stay on both these prescriptions until I was in my mid to late twenties. Was it any wonder I wasn't able to conceive being messed about with by medication from such a young age?

The pain grew much worse in adulthood; I ended up in A&E three times as I had passed out in the street or office. Not much sympathy with the medical staff there, just a painkiller and "it's just period pains, you need to be tougher about it, it comes every month deal with it." Mostly male doctors, but a few female ones too. I felt shamed.

After the initial chart with the smear nurse, I opted in for some further investigation. I first had a vaginal examination followed by an internal ultrasound scan. They found endometriosis, so I was booked for a laparoscopy to be sure this was the diagnosis; this is where the surgeon makes incisions in your stomach instead of creating a whacking great big hole across your groin then sewing you up. Neat. Once this was confirmed, I started my first course of laser treatment to blast away the endometriosis where they could. Endometriosis is where the endometrial lining of the womb grows in other areas like the fallopian tubes or ovaries. It can be extremely painful during your period, making those days worse with even heavier bleeding; it can cause pain in sex, extreme fatigue, difficulty getting pregnant, and depression from long-term pain. For a while, I believed the scans, surgery, and laser treatment had worked, as my monthly agony had all but disappeared. For a while at least.

·····

I grew up a Catholic and went to an all-girls private school where we went to church at least three times a week and we were definitely made to pray every day in classes. So that fact that I had once been pregnant, unplanned, of course, made me feel like I had committed a cardinal sin.

I was twenty-six and when I found out I was pregnant. I knew I wanted to be a mother, but still, I had never given it much thought other than that; I mean, I had grown up on the pill. My then non-committal, don't make the mistake of even leaving a toothbrush in his flat, boyfriend absolutely did not want a family. In fact, it was the beginning of the demise of that relationship, unsurprisingly. The family members I had confided in did not think I was ready to handle being a mother either and being highly emotional and easily swayed, I found myself booked into a Marie Stopes clinic in London.

I went on my own, the 'boyfriend' was too busy with his very important meetings at his very important job to be with me, his *not* very important girlfriend. It was decided not to give me a general anaesthetic, just a local; I am not sure why I was never consulted. *Just ask them why? I can't. I don't want to be a nuisance and ask; I was probably just another young woman stupid enough to stuff her life up with an unwanted pregnancy.* The catholic faith started slipping into my internal monologue. Anyway, they were professionals, so I just blindly trusted them.

I felt every part of that procedure, or it seemed that way. I was paralysed with pain and fear on the operating table, tears flowing from my eyes, rendering me mute for hours afterwards as I had buried myself deep within to survive it. I felt such shame sitting in the bath back at home some hours later post procedure the hot water tinged with red, weeping silently in pain, grief swallowing me up, and shivering uncontrollably with the shock of it all. I stepped out of the bath and shoved down the trauma, stuffing it into my mental baggage to unpack when I felt stronger. Two days later, I was admitted to Chelsea and Westminster Hospital as a fever had taken hold of my body, riddled with fear, shame, and I was doubled over in pain. I was hooked up to an IV as the infection had jumped in on top of the grief. Stayed there for three days, staring out the dirty window at London feeling more than foolish. It turned out I was miscarrying parts the surgeons at the clinic had missed.

So yeah, deep down, I knew it would be me; I have always held a notion from those old Catholic school days that I would be punished for that abortion. Nonetheless, the medical professionals continued to poke and prod, drew countless amounts of blood, injected my ovaries with blue dye that caused me to pass out from the pain that felt like I had been stabbed. All this to find out why I can't conceive. I've had too many speculums and swabs inserted to bother counting them anymore. *Dignity? What dignity – that ran screaming from the building the time I had to spread my legs into stirrups and allow eight young male doctor students all have a gander to play a game of 'guess what's wrong with this uterus?'*

Once the tests were done and the results in, the anxiety started to step up a few gears, and being used to stuffing the truth down, I ignored how my self-loathing was gathering speed and we continued on regardless. *How bloody British of me!*

It was not just me they tested, but Henri too. His sperm needed to be counted and viewed under a microscope to see if there was a problem there. I don't think Henri was prepared for his part in the testing rigmarole we were going through. A sort of denial had crept in, so when his day arrived, his stress levels were pushed to maximum. He was holed up in our bathroom trying to get a sample whilst I waited impatiently downstairs.

I am guessing I wasn't very helpful when I shouted up the stairs every few minutes, checking on how he was getting on. The pressure meant it took a very long time but he adamantly, absolutely, did not want my help. Fair enough.

Finally, success, the sample secured, and our thirty-minute window to do the hospital dash, keeping that sample as warm as possible, had begun. Simple. We were twenty minutes away. What could go wrong with ten minutes to spare?

Well, tractors, for starters. Two of them in tandem, pulling out in front of us, trundling along at the top speed of twenty miles an hour. *Bollocks. Just our luck.* They finally turned off, but before I could put my foot down to make up time, we came upon an accident forcing us to divert to the longer route round. The clock was ticking. *Tick. Tick.*

City Centre traffic was as standard, but by now, we were already delayed. Then, when we thought all was lost, an open road lay ahead so I didn't hesitate to accelerate to try and make up time. Just as we thought we were making up for some time, an L-plated car pulled out of a hidden driveway on a bend. Not just a learner driver but one having trouble changing gears, bunny hopping all over the place, making our tyres make that awful screeching sound and jerking us to an almost stop, at which point Henri lost his grip on his sample. "Shit!" In slow motion (as if we were in a rom-com movie), we watched as it somersaulted into the air. It landed on my lap, so I shoved it between my legs for warmth and overtook the learner driver in one swift move. I would like to say that I made this manoeuvre safely but the fact that Henri had his nails embedded in the dashboard with his eyes squeezed shut indicates perhaps not. *Tick. Tick.*

At twenty-eight minutes exactly, I pulled to a stop outside the main hospital doors. Henri leapt from the car, leaving the door hanging open and ran as fast as he could to the third floor to deliver our precious cargo.

Tick. Tick. Boom.

My own tests were all negative or unexplained. I was formally diagnosed with endometriosis, which I already knew, adenomyosis (where the endometrial lining of the womb grows into the muscular wall) and endometrioma (a cyst filled with chocolate-looking type sauce). *Mmm, yummy.*

Lucky me, a trio that was responsible for crippling my body two weeks of every month. All of which would miraculously disappear when I get pregnant, apparently. A new appointment was made to plan some laparoscopic surgery for another good rummage around, followed by some more laser work to try and banish the endometriosis and see if that helped clear things up a bit more. As if I had a cold. Henri's swimmers were good, some swimming the wrong way, but they were up for the job, presumably once they had worked out how to turn around.

What came next was not more medical procedures or hospital visits but our delayed honeymoon; a three-week trip starting with four days in New York, another four days in Miami, and the remaining time in Jamaica. What a gloriously decadent trip of a lifetime that was. Shopping and sightseeing in an uber cool and cosmopolitan city, soaking up the party atmosphere in a warmer, more tropical city, before swimming daily in the sea and an infinity pool, eating fresh fish and an abundance of the sweetest fruits, and discovering the delights of a well-made pina colada!

A trip we very much needed at the right time, a true break from the hum drum of every day, from anxiety that had set up lodgings in my head. Above all, overflowing with love and happiness, a carefree existence. Buckets of smiling, sunshine, laughter, just being us again with no pressures from the life we had left behind for a while.

Pregnant Pause

We came home from that trip surprised that we were pregnant, relaxed, and happier than we'd ever been; such was the miracle of new life inside me. I didn't know we were pregnant as we landed on English soil, but a few weeks later, I suspected as I calculated I was at least three weeks late for my period, confirmed by a pee-on-a-stick test. I wanted to wait to be sure so booked an appointment to see a doctor.

It was a summer's morning; I was not working until after lunch, so I decided a long walk across the fields with Digby out for his daily walk would be pretty. Bending to unleash his lead in a field, a dull thud started to pulse in my lower back; I stretched and popped away any negative thought bubbles. Reaching home, I kicked my trainers off at the door and wriggled out of my sweatshirt that was stuck to me from the sweat, a combination of the early summer heat, a quickened pace to get home, and pure fear that was dancing in my chest. "No, no, no. Please no." I threw myself on the old, soft sofa in the conservatory and Digby jumped up next to me, resting his head on my lap as he had become accustomed to doing. As I lay there, the thudding pain dulled to nothing, I felt stronger to climb the stairs to get out of these sweaty clothes and to the bathroom. I needed to make sure there was no blood in my pants. As I sat down on the toilet, a searing, red-hot pain ripped through me, bringing with it fresh, bright red blood. The pain took hold with such a fierce rage that within a few hours, I knew our early miracle pregnancy had abruptly ended.

Any unbridled joy I had felt was ripped away in an instant, including robbing me of any special moments with Henri, let alone family and friends. I had kept it from family to be one hundred per cent sure, a doctor's appointment booked to confirm it.

I kept the appointment and told them what had happened, only to be referred back to my consultant and told to try and get on with my life.

The questions that come with a miscarriage are brutal, *what did I do wrong? What could I have done to prevent it? This is all my fault. Again. What is wrong with my body? Why? WHY?* Of course, I never did anything wrong; there was no preventing it. It was just not meant to be, and accepting this fact took us both a lot of time. The tiny shard of hope it did give us was that I could get pregnant. Maybe then. Just maybe.

As we slowly recovered into the winter months, conversations about the possibility of adopting began. A simple internet search and the figures were plain to see, so many children living life alone or with a foster family as they were taken from their parents; adults that should have known better. Reading the statistics made for heartbreak which in turn cemented our decision to make a difference to at least one child. We pressed buttons to start the process and booked in for an information session. On the morning we were due to go, we woke up to see there had been a heavy snowfall overnight, the first time in years we'd seen any snow at all, let alone that much of it, preventing us getting there or anywhere in fact. I tried to rearrange several times, but they were vague and dismissive, and the whole thing became very frustrating. We shelved it, putting it down as the wrong time for us as around the same time, we were offered in vitro fertilisation (in simple terms, this is medically assisted pregnancy) by our gynae consultant doctor on the condition I tried a drug called Clomid first.

Our consultation for that prescription appointment was short but ended with the doctor giving Henri a lighthearted warning that he needed to "hide all the sharp objects in case aggression takes hold, although there is a chance you may be one of the lucky few who don't get any side effects from this drug. Let's see where the chips fall." *O how we laughed. Such a* *joker. *eye roll** Looking back now, I hope doctors have become more respectful and tactful, not just in how that throwaway comment was directed at the male in the relationship but how that strengthened my own self-loathing.

Clomid is a medication that could aid a natural conception; it is an anti-estrogen, non-steroidal medicine to aid with fertility. The drug is supposed to kick-start the pituitary gland to release hormones that are needed to stimulate ovulation. The small print tells you that it makes you hot, gives you nausea, headaches, stomach cramps, painful periods, weight gain, bloated belly, and dark spots can form in front of your eyes affecting vision. Sounds fun, right? I had it all; of course I did. What the small print doesn't tell you is that it twists your personality. I went from a mostly happy, emotional wreck trying to keep it all together to a raging bull with no filter, absolutely not keeping it together. I could not contain the fire inside me; I screamed and shouted like I was the only one that mattered, I cried a lot, I even punched a wall in an explosive, violent anger-driven moment. I was hideous to live with.

The kicker came when, one Sunday as I was cooking a roast dinner, we were both ravenous after skipping breakfast and working in our garden. When the roasting timer went off and I went to put the meal together, I realised I hadn't turned the oven on in the first place and, therefore, nothing had roasted. In a flash, a full-on instant rage consumed me, I slammed the oven door shut as hard as I could, picked up the nearest item that was in reach, which happened to be that aforementioned sharp object and I hurled it as hard as I could at the wall. I turned and flew up the stairs, screaming obscenities before burying my head in pillows on the bed. It is fair to say I was hysterical, hanger at its absolute worst. I wish I could say I was exaggerating.

That was the end of my Clomid trial. I never took another one of those pills again. No one deserves to go through that or live with it. It took around a month for me to return back to my normal, calmer self, but we were still no further forward.

Part Two
The IVF years

In Vitro Fertilisation

Ask anyone about In Vitro Fertilisation, your friends, an aunt, the neighbours, work colleagues or even your local greengrocer and I will be willing to bet they know someone (like their best friend's aunt's daughter) that has had a successful pregnancy from going through the IVF process. Usually, these conversations will end with, "Ooo I wonder if you will have twins or even triplets! Imagine that!" but never, "What happens if it doesn't work"?

IVF not working is never really spoken about, like it's taboo in some way. There seems to be this innate thought process that IVF is the saving grace to any couple not being able to conceive naturally. Think back to any of the IVF stories you have ever heard, and the headlines are usually dominated with something along the lines of '...and they all lived happily ever after as a family of three or four.' Well, not quite, but you catch my drift. In principle, IVF is generally perceived as a success story in the main, a miracle procedure that produces a baby even to those who had to try nine times.

Personally, I know of three couples in the last six months that IVF has worked its magic for. One on the first round of IVF and her second successful IVF pregnancy, another couple, a cautious but successful walk through it for the second time after a failed first attempt and the last couple, after seven tries, have just had an adorable baby girl. It is quite wonderful when it works.

When we first started, we rode the wave of positivity, believing it was surely our turn for success.

Henri and I made the decision to be open about our IVF journey with our friends and family. We felt we could be better supported this way and not have to pile all that pressure on ourselves and implode from the stress of it. Giving ourselves permission to have outlets to relieve our frustrations other than just inside our mini two-person (and a dog) circle. Share the load, so to speak.

My mother spent her days cutting IVF success stories out of the newspaper, my father did not want to talk about it or even acknowledge it for that matter, my sister was quietly hopeful, and my friends asked little to no questions at all. Not quite the support we were expecting. In fact, it took a while for me to register, but mostly, the people we loved and spent time with started to go quiet on us. We got it; it's a delicate subject to approach. They didn't want to upset us or say the wrong thing, so they thought it best to say nothing at all. We understood it was too much pressure for them, for our friendships, so we remained on our little island, holding each other up.

That said, though, once we had confided in a few people, the word spread around our small circle of friends; people knew of our plight, which meant that some people would see us and relay how their friend's friend or cousin or colleague had IVF and how now they have a little girl or boy or twins. It was well-meaning but added to our nerves and eventually the weight of our failures. Everyone seemed to have a positive story to tell or advice to impart. That or the topic of children just never came up.

Some friends decided that they would not share their own good news that a beautiful bouncing bundle of joy was on the way; as if this happy news may upset us, they carried the baby guiltily because we could not. News flash, not telling us was way more hurtful especially when we bump into you months later pushing a pram in a supermarket. Again, I sort of get that it is awkward; I do, but we are friends surely that means we share our good and bad news. It just made us feel alienated further.

Our starter consultation was at the main hospital, in the pregnancy unit. As we sat down excited to start, I looked around the waiting room, the walls covered in peeling pastel green paint, some areas patched over with pregnancy posters. Cold, uncomfortable blue plastic seats followed the line of the walls, a noisy glugging water machine breaking the hushed silence and a table adorned with pregnancy magazines to peruse as you wait. Midwives wafted in and out, calling the names of their pregnant patients; we were the only ones waiting in that room without a protruding belly. I felt like I stuck out like Belisha Beacon. Had I, in fact, walked into the wrong waiting room? Anxiety kicked in hard, and I was struggling to breathe normally, loud, muddled thoughts flooding my brain rushing in all at once. My mind snapped out of its downward trajectory as our names were called by our allocated midwife as she introduced herself to us. The relief of a smiling, friendly face was felt by us both; we smiled back, took a breath, held hands, and stood to start our new chapter - one that we hoped was going to have that happy ever-after ending.

It is a funny thing when you start a journey like IVF; you fill yourself with so much unsullied hope, all those success stories, the miracle babies. We had an absolute belief that this would work. Why wouldn't it? We walked away from that initial appointment excited, on cloud nine and eager to start. We had been taught how to inject a needle into my stomach or thigh, talked about what to expect from each part of the procedure, been handed a timescale chart for different medications starting at different times, and a what not to do list noted down in our heads. The drive home was an excited, happy babble of conversations about our future family life. All we needed to do now was wait for the arrival of the meds from a courier they had organised. *We have a plan. A real tangible plan.*

Life continued. We worked. We went out. We worked out. We walked Digby and planned a holiday. One frosty morning in the spring the box of medication arrived in a cooler box, and its arrival made us stop in our tracks. *It is actually happening;*

the meds are making this real. Wow, so many different drugs. We made room in the fridge by clearing an entire shelf and counting the days down until we arrived at day one. We needed to wait for the right time in my monthly cycle. Just before we began, we did the obligatory pregnancy test to be sure we were not, in fact, pregnant. Pregnancy tests have become my nemesis these days; they always end in disappointment. This one was no different.

Never have I felt more nervous, more mentally unequipped, more pressure than on the morning of day one, but we were ready to start. Together, we filled the vial up with the clear liquid medication, sat on the end of our bed in silence. We looked at each other in silence and the sting of tears started to fill my eyes.

"Are you ready? This is so weird." I nodded, letting the tears flow from my eyes and he shakily inserted the needle into my stomach and just like that IVF had started. It really had come to this.

There was no fanfare or cheer. Quite an underwhelming moment.

The first lot of meds were to quieten my body, take it from a stormy sea to a quiet lake, stopping all activity in my womb. When the meds kicked in a few days later, it was like I could hear my body for the first time in years. My mind became a sanctuary and I found I could sit with my thoughts easier. I was calm. It felt strange not to be so chaotic with my thoughts. It was a good place to be. This mental state was the way I wanted to live; my anxiety was barely audible.

Then, we switched it up as per the instruction chart. These new meds woke my cycle up with a bang, stimulating the follicles, pushing my ovaries to make eggs, lots of them and big ones. Eggs they hoped were going to be strong enough to withstand the force of this process. The whoosh of my mind cranked up and the sanctuary I was enjoying demolished within days of the new drugs kicking into my system. Starting back with headaches, the noise came back, and the pain too. My chest once again heavy and tight.

For three weeks, we injected my stomach at the same time every morning, by week three my belly looked like it had been punched repeatedly, sporting an assortment of colours, black, purple, blue, with hues of orange and green, our constant physical IVF evidence. My belly resembled a piece of modern art that makes no sense except to us. I was starting to swell too. So sore to touch and uncomfortable in a way I had never felt before. Clothes began tightening at the seams as I bloated a little more each day. My breasts were so tender, and the fatigue made getting through the day feel like walking on the beach in six-inch stilettos, such an effort. The last week of injections, my emotions were on a rollercoaster, one day up, another down. We finally made it to scan day where we were to see if the eggs were big enough to be surgically harvested. They were not, so we spent another ten days injecting some more, but this time, we had moved the injection site to the inner thigh, so a new pattern of bruising was starting to form. I could no longer wear anything other than an elasticated tracksuit as my stomach had ironically grown to look like I was five months pregnant. The irony was certainly not lost on us. It occurred to me that this was yet another cruel twist in this bizarre journey, of course no baby but huge ovaries the size of small melons carrying eggs at abnormal sizes. This stage of IVF is, in fact, quite perilous; they call it OHSS, ovarian hyperstimulation syndrome. As it suggests, the ovaries become overstimulated, which potentially brings with it blood clotting, kidney failure and fluid buildup in the belly and into the lungs. Lovely, just one more added to the list for anxiety to get in a tizzy about.

Extraction or egg removal day is here, I feel like a beached whale at this point, so I am really ready to go under general anesthetic to have these eggs harvested. Henri and I barely spoke to each other the morning before the operation, both of us living in our own heads, just following the instructions of the nurses on duty. I certainly appeared calm, but inside I was a jellified mess. Had the eggs grown large enough? My swollen belly would have yelled yes if it could speak; I was at bursting point and ridiculously uncomfortable. Part of me worried more about the next steps, the other part unable to wait another hour as the pain of being so huge had become almost unbearable. *Stick a fork in me, I am done.*

Our hospital is mostly a lovely, warm place to be, but the women's unit is in the old wing, which means drafty corridors constructed from concrete blocks. It appears as if it was once a pathway leading around the red brick building and then it was decided to build walls on the edge of the path, with a tin roof to hold the rain at bay, adding holes for windows (although there was an absence of glass in those holes) thus creating a corridor to the building. Footsteps and voices echo off the drab, bare walls, giving it quite an eerie feel, especially when the cold wind howls through it. Once inside the red brick building, the décor feels a little like you've stepped into the war hospital from the 1940s. Nothing much has been updated, I suspect, since it had been built. The staff, though, are the opposite, warm, kind, and gentle with their hands.

With lots of reassurance, I was in and out of surgery there very quickly. They managed to retrieve eight beautiful big eggs within twenty minutes. I felt like a proud mother hen.

Whilst I was blissfully unaware of anything happening, Henri was shown to a small room, apparently not unlike the size of a coat cupboard. It housed a hard plastic (wipeable) seat and a small also plastic table with some top shelf, seen-better-days, porn magazines piled on it, a tissue box, and a bin. He clutched the sample tub he had been given whilst the nurse instructed him to do 'his business'. *Sexy.*

It felt exhausting that morning, but we headed home knowing that in the lab by the smaller car park the medical professionals were busy making our babies. My eggs meeting

Henri's sperm. Time to wait. We would be called in the morning.

A sleepless night led to a fretful morning; around mid-morning, the consultant called us to say they had successfully made four embryos, and these were splitting nicely; he expected to see progress in the next twenty-four hours. *It's working! All of this is working!* We were not even nearly there, but this news was good news and we allowed ourselves to roll around in it.

Twenty-four hours later, two of the embryos had survived and split and they were ready to be transferred into my womb. Disappointed that we had nothing to freeze, but this round would work; it had worked for everybody else's best friend's neighbour's daughter. It had to work. We deserved it to work.

Back to the hospital we went. Anyone observing us would see a couple smiling, arm in arm. A hopeful young couple happily in love. We walked in step with each other, holding each other up. The embryo transfer was swift, and we watched on the monitor as our embryos were embedded into the lining of my womb. *There they are, alive inside me.* Technically, this made me pregnant. Two weeks it would take to get the embryos to nestle in comfortably. Just two weeks. I was advised to rest with no exercise, and in fourteen days, a pregnancy test will confirm it all. Simple.

Turns out two weeks is a very, very long time. I am an Italian Scorpio, so patience is not a strong character trait. The first week, I did absolutely nothing. I sat on the couch all day. I was lazy and loved it to start with, with no work, no commitments. I would read for hours, watch endless episodes of Supernatural, and stare wistfully into the open fire, dreaming of what our little family would look like. I took the prescribed rest notice very seriously. However, by week two, I was bored of doing the sum total of nothing, but happily imagining the embryos nestling inside my warm, all cosy and safe, so I guess despite the boredom, so far, so good. I slowly and gently walked Digby around the village and started cooking again for us, a reprieve from the convenience meals that tasted all the same. I turned to Google for hours at a time, learning about the 'two-week wait,' discovering lots of forums of women in the same place I was. Waiting. So many forums, so many women. I skim-read it all, stopping only to read all the faceless success stories. *What am I doing?* Willing my mind to believe everything was as it should be and in four days, I would be peeing on that test stick and it would be positive. I was gathering speed in my anticipation and the idea of it was growing large in my mind. Together, Henri and I had hope. When you have hope and feel so positive, how can it go wrong?

Day twelve of fourteen and Henri went to work planting a kiss on my forehead, telling me to rest some more. I settle myself down on the sofa; by this point, I am quite surprised there is not a bottom-shaped indent in the cushioned seat I have sat down so much. Deciding I need a distraction, I want to carry on with my knitting project of a little blanket for our baby in a soft pale yellow. Realising I had left the needles upstairs by the bed, I start the climb the stairs, noting that I am feeling sluggish. I am midway up and I stop. Something is wrong. I feel a wetness in my pants. I rush up the rest of the stairs, taking two at a time and bolt into the bathroom, pulling at my clothes and I sit on the toilet. I take a breath before looking down and there it is. Fresh blood resting on the gusset. I wipe and there is some more, but not a huge amount. The panic is rising from my stomach to my chest. Pain rips through it and I know I am having a panic attack. Standing to get more air in my lungs, I grip the sides of the sink and look in the mirror, forcing myself to breathe and stay calm. I am shaking. I stare straight into my own dark blue eyes; I see they are frightened. Could this be the end?

As soon as I am able, I find my phone and call the hospital to explain what's happening. They ask me to take a test straight away. I do.

....

Years ago, I remember taking a pregnancy test in the beautiful mountain town of Verbier in Switzerland. I was skiing with friends of my boyfriend, who did not feel I was important enough to fly with me, he had work to finish, so I flew with them. I felt sick all the time, so eating was the last thing on my mind, I could not face the wine, it smelt so bad, and I was completely exhausted. I thought I had flu. I confided in one of the girlfriends there that I vaguely knew from a different past. She suggested I was pregnant, and she laughed at the ridiculousness of me potentially being pregnant with *his* baby. She laughed so hard I wanted to punch her in the face. All the while thinking she may have a point, I bought a test and took it back to the chalet to pee and wait the required five minutes for the result. Positive. I did another. Positive. Positive. Positive. Four tests are laid out before me.

I dial his number. No reply, but then a text message saying he was busy; what did I want? I did not reply. I lay on the bed and cried, putting a hand on my belly. A baby. Pulling on some warm clothes I snuck out to avoid the 'what was the result, what was I going to do' questions that would be fired at me and went for a walk in the cold, dusky, late afternoon. Snow-covered mountains with the sun penetrating the low clouds gave the town a sparkle, like glitter had been sprinkled all over it. I breathed in and told my belly everything would be ok.

He finally found time to call, and I picked up and told him. Fury. That was his response. He was furious and I was instantly transported back to childhood, feeling like I had really landed myself in trouble. He said he was flying out tomorrow we would talk then. "I want to talk now. I really feel

I just need to map out an initial plan. I am worried about skiing in case I fall and hurt the baby."

"Plan? Ok here's the plan, I fly in tomorrow, we holiday and then we go home, and we will get rid of it." He hung up. I am sorry I lied, baby; I was not strong enough.

••••••••••

I called Henri and tell him that there was blood and a test declared it was negative. It is the end. We are not pregnant. All our hopes and dreams crash around us, smashing into tiny little pieces and both our hearts break at the same time.

Unlike all the other men to have entered my life he stops what he is doing and comes home to be with me.

We Go Again

After our first IVF failed, I was crushed; I wanted to pull our duvet over my head and stay there in the dark and cry. Shut the world out. Pull in Henri and Digby and maybe live under there for a while, cosy under the sheets in the dark. *I was so sure we would be successful. How could this have possibly gone wrong?* I had convinced myself it would work. I had listened to all the triumphant stories even though I had tried so hard not to. The hope we held was like a balloon; the more I heard a success story, the closer we got to the transfer, the more I did each day as the doctors asked me to, the more the balloon kept filling up with air.

POP!

We overfilled it; we killed the vibe.

Our consultant dismissed our first failed foray into IVF with a waft of his hand saying, "We go again."

We had 'won' three rounds of IVF on the NHS. In some counties across the UK, it is only one or two. We were lucky, especially given our age, I am told. In the first appointment with our consultant, I asked why the hospitals granted only a few tries and, in some cases, just one.

"Well, honestly, childless couples are not in a life-or-death situation. This is the allocation of budget that is deemed acceptable."

I argued back (*I know, shocker!),* "Not being able to have a family naturally leads to mental health issues or even depression, and in some people, surely the balance of life and death is real for them without fulfilling their dreams. At least it can *feel* like that."

Our consultant looked me dead in the eye, and without sugar-coating it said, "How would you feel if the monies were allocated to you and a very ill person, say, with cancer, was told there was no money left in the pot because it all went on couples needing IVF. There must be a cutoff point."

How do you respond to that sucker punch? Such is the UK's healthcare lottery. I carried that conversation on with Henri in the car after our appointment complaining and moaning that "we have never once claimed for benefits or asked for government handouts. This is our thing, surely it is ok not to feel guilty that we are trying to have children." My statement hung in the air like a bad smell. Not content with my body not working as it should, now I was so desperate I was scraping the barrel with justification for our treatment. We never really spoke about it again, but now I look back on it, and I toy with how selfish I would have been if it hadn't been capped at three rounds. Did someone really suffer because we took some NHS budget for IVF? IVF that didn't even work. Money spent on us, wasted that could have saved someone's life. I think I will always carry some guilt with me.

Within a few weeks, we had a new delivery of medication arrive at our door. I was asked by the same delivery guy to sign for them. He couldn't meet my eye. He knew our secret and it was awkward. Maybe it was just me that was awkward. As I saw it, he knew I was the woman who had a womb that was defunct, that we needed to try again; that was enough for me to *be* awkward.

We stepped back on the merry-go-round and started injecting into the leftover blush of old bruises. Everything was the same, the calm followed by the storm.

This time, I had developed enough mature eggs to have them retrieved earlier than in previous cycles. The consultant was very happy with this round. My body, he said, was learning. The transfer was smooth and before I knew it, I was back at home in the same seat on the sofa with two weeks of waiting ahead of me. This time though, I was not excited, this time, all I felt was panic. Gripped within its grasp. It constricted my throat, cast pain into my abdomen, made me dizzy, and my heart literally felt heavy.

It was as if I already knew the outcome. Day three and the bleeding started, and it didn't stop. It got heavier and heavier, and we knew it was over once more.

I cried. Rivers of tears, lakes, and oceans. I felt like my body was giving up, my body was done, and my mind was following. I was in full grief mode. I have lost another child, four times now. I needed a break. Just a small interlude before putting myself back in the ring. Day after day, I sat on that sofa by the fire all day, just staring at the flickering flames. Healing this time was unhurried. Slowly I started to allow myself to go back to walking Digby and basic household functions whilst Henri was at work. I spoke to no one. I had no interest in speaking to anyone. I even ordered the food shop online. I ventured nowhere. I needed time.

In a checkup with my GP, he indicated I needed to see a therapist, so he referred me to the waiting list. The list for mental health was longer than I anticipated; a full eight months before I could see someone. Once again, I was not a priority because I was not suicidal. It was not life or death. Whilst that is true, I was, however, at rock bottom, I was on my knees asking for help from the bottom of a dark, uncomfortably hard well. I did not know how to climb out.

One Sunday, a few months after our second loss, we were cuddled on the sofa, a roaring fire in the hearth and a movie on the TV. Digby lay at our feet, gently snoring. It was cold and wet outside; the wind was furious. My phone pinged through with a message notification. It was from my friend Molly, I had not heard from her in a long time. The last time I had seen her, we were about to start IVF number one, drinking cocktails in London, where we confided in each other about our family-making woes. Molly had done a random fertility test that she had bought discounted as an afterthought when scrolling for deals on Wowcher and it did not turn out as she had hoped. In fact, she had no hint that anything was wrong. She needed to start Clomid, potentially then venturing into IVF too. As selfish as this sounds, I was equally sad for her, knowing what lay ahead and delighted I had someone on a similar path to me. Finally, someone may understand where we were at, we could support each other through it. We hugged a lot and cried a little.

Her message flashed at me, so I picked up the phone and read.

"Hey you! Gosh long time no speak – it has been a while hasn't it! Soz not responded to your texts recently it has just been sooooo busy. Anyway, I have news. I am up the duff!! Bit of a fucker really as it means we can't go skiing. Thought you would like to know! Chat soon. Lots of love."

I did want to know, of course I did.

Up the duff. Bit of a fucker. Can't go skiing. Been so busy. Bit of a fucker.

The tears rolled and they didn't stop. I quickly became hysterical. I was angry. Henri read the message. He said nothing but tried to pull me into a hug. I pushed him away. Hard. I started to scream.

"BIT OF A FUCKER. CAN'T GO SKIING! I WOULD LOVE TO HAVE TO CANCEL SKIING BECAUSE I'M PREGNANT OR SHOULD I SAY UP THE FUCKING DUFF."

I shouted and shouted and ugly cried, snot coming from my nose, spittle firing out of my mouth. My head felt like it was going to explode. By this point, I was standing, the dog was barking concern, Henri was on his feet trying to calm me down. One last huge scream and I collapsed on the floor. Lifeless like the babies I didn't have growing inside me. Not an ounce of energy left. Quietly sobbing now. Digby licking my tears and my husband rubbing my back and we stayed that way for hours. It was dark when I allowed him to pull me up to bed.

It really was not until very recently that I came to acknowledge that losing an IVF round at twelve days, three days or nine days comes under baby loss. Not to be confused with miscarriage – that is different. They may have been minuscule, but a failed IVF is a loss. It carries weight in your heart and totting up all my losses means that I have, in fact, in my lifetime lost six babies that I am aware of.

Once More Unto The Breach

After I broke apart, it took a while, but the light started to seep back in through the fissures that grief had created; my pain laid bare as a china cup would look if it had crashed onto a thinly carpeted floor, nearly shattering into pieces but strangely held together despite the obvious cracks running through it. Together, our family of three took long walks in the woods, tramped across wet, muddy fields, and drove down to the coast to taste the salty air and breathe with the rhythm of the waves. The air and nature soothed us, wrapped us up until a calm descended. Our solitary togetherness strengthened our existing bonds. Spring arrived once more and with the pops of colour sprouting from the ground, birds taking baths and splashing in the puddles left over from rain showers, lush green fields filling up with bleating lambs, and pink blossoms floating down from all the trees, buds of fresh hope.

We contacted the consultant to say we were ready for our last spin of the wheel in IVF. We had to join the waitlist, which was approximately five weeks long.

Whilst waiting for the next round of IVF, we got to work on modernising our 1850s house. We needed a new roof, so we scraped together the money for that. Then the pond had to go as Digby had been caught too many times taking a dip in the smelly pond water swimming. Hard no. So, we filled it in, sourcing stone for the patio to come from around the same era as the house was built. It felt fitting. We knocked one side of the garage down to build a more modern carport. In the orchard, we used old railway sleepers to make three raised beds, added a greenhouse too. Our gardening skills were not much cop for such a mature garden and a massive orchard full of fruit trees, so we hired a gardener at an extortionate rate per hour. It was a necessary spend, we were drowning in plants, weeds and out-of-control brambles. A small part of a wall downstairs in the hallway was looking like there could be mould there or more precisely rot, something like that coming through. All this work forced us to take a look at our finances versus how hard we were working and what we still needed to fix. Something needed to change. We were both earning good money, but our hours were long, relentless, and our house felt like a drain on all our hard work. Our beautiful dream home had become a noose around our neck.

We knew we needed to move. I yearned to be nearer to my family in Dorset. Wiltshire, as beautiful as it was, it was not giving us the support we needed. My father mentioned quite out of the blue that we could live in one of his apartments in my old hometown. Shall we move? Could we? Should we? Shall we just go for it? How would Henri's business work? Mine, well I could just stop. It was a service-led business and frankly, I had had enough of demanding clients taking me for granted and staff that didn't want to work besides, all I wanted to do was to write and be a mother.

I shrugged, "Ok. Let's just go and have a look. There could be an opportunity to open a barbershop there, we could sell our existing shop and just have it all in one place. You've stormed it here, why can't you create a new shop there with just as much success? There's the direct train too, although that will probably cost a bit. We need to do something, get rid of this financial burden."

"You are right, financially, we cannot carry on this way. It is like we have a money leak and no way to plug it. I say yes, let's see it."

We took the train from the city station on a sunny Sunday and went to see the apartment. It was not a standard apartment, as it turned out. Built around 1660, the walls were sturdy and thick. It boasted three levels, sat above an Indian restaurant. Its neighbours, two pubs right in the heart of Sherborne. The entrance hall was modest and small but an iron spiral staircase to the left took you up to the first floor. A patio door led to a private balcony above the courtyard below, the doorway directly in front of the staircase led to an enormous kitchen, which in turn led to the bathroom and more steps up, this time wooden, taking you to a big room in the eaves. Back at the top of the spiral staircase were four steps leading to a hallway; to the left was a large bedroom, in front a smaller room currently being used as a study and finally to the right a huge sitting room, all with distinctly high ceilings and giant, impressive sash windows. All three of these rooms looked out onto the splendour of an old Abbey. There was work to be done. The bathroom needed to be gutted, and the windows needed to be taken out and replaced with double glazing. There was no heating, no boiler in fact, no fireplace. It needed new carpets with the thickest underlay to block out the sounds of Indian music floating up, as the current ones looked threadbare and browner than their original colour. It needed more than a lick of paint but also a family to love it. All doable. No massive garden, mouldy wall, or leaking roof.

On our train ride home, there was excitement in our chatter that was awash with ideas and plans for our future. We were animated for the first time in so long. Such is the effect of something else to look forward to too, which was not lost on either of us. We were going to move. We needed to do this.

Planning began and so did round three of IVF. *Ding ding!*

Between the injections we worked hard, sorting through our huge amount of collected (some would say hoarded) stuff over the years. Both of us are hoarders of a sort, so our work was cut out for us. Downsizing from a four-bedroomed house with a garage full of bits and bobs. In the orchard, the long wooden building that was at least twenty feet by eight feet housed gardening tools and stacks of furniture we didn't need handed down from my father's own downsizing. He had a few years back turned up unannounced with a lorry full of furniture for us to have (even though we did not need it) as he went from a five-bedroomed house to an apartment. With nowhere to put it, we shoved it into this building. It was our problem now. There was an enormous amount to do. Both of us were occupied, which helped us move forward through the IVF cycle of injecting, bruising, swelling. Rooms were looking clearer, ready for photographs for our white house to go on the market.

Transfer number three was nearly upon us. One last week of injecting. It was this week that the house went on the market. We sold the house within three days. *Wait. What?* We were both stunned that it took no time at all. The agent told us we needed to move fast as they wanted to be in within three weeks. Three weeks. So, we needed to pack up an entire house, find a removals company, make sure the other place was empty and at least clean, but more importantly, we would be inside our final two weeks' wait. I was not supposed to do anything during that time let alone pack a house up, lift heavy objects and move home.

We hired packers and movers. *Tick.* Went to clean up our new home. *Tick.* The transfer happened in a blink. *Tick.* I even hired a cleaner to clean our sold house. *Tick.* Anticipation of demanding pushy buyers. *FAIL.* Our buyers wanted to push the move forward by another week or they threatened to pull out, asking for so many visits to measure for curtains and furniture, they called the agent wanting the garden cleared of certain plants and trees before they moved in, they brought around builders and tradesmen. It was chaotic.

There was not a minute to even think about googling the forums and obsessing over the details of what was happening inside me. I felt like I was a ball of stress. Imagine Mr Messy from the Mr Men. That. Henri was the same. Digby had no idea what was going on.

Move day arrived and with it a trickle of blood. *No. No. No. It is day nine. No. Please no.* The movers were with us at 6am and the cleaner at 11am cleaning around the movers. It was muddled. I needed to help out as time was running out, the new owners were due in a few hours and still so much to do. The bleeding stopped. *Breathe Loretta. You have got this. Just a few more rooms to clear and then in the car away to a new way of living, a slower pace.*

Upstairs in our empty bedroom, I surveyed the room. I silently said goodbye to all the memories this room held. Under the window where Chloe, our 19-year-old cat died, the accidental discovery of an old enormous fireplace, injecting on the bed for the first time, all the times. Henri got down on one knee in here with a ring threaded through the last rose in the garden to propose on my birthday because he knew I dreaded birthdays, and he wanted me to always celebrate the day. All the learning and growing we did here.

I bent to pick up a protective floor cover the movers had left behind. As I came back up, I was thrown forward by a pain in my lower back so sharp it took the breath from my body. I fell on my knees, waiting for the pain to subside. It did not. It gathered speed. I felt a hot flush between my legs. Blood. I did not even need to look. The pain shifted to my groin, gripping my whole body. Tears sprung from my eyes. This time around, I was not sad; I was angry. So angry. Why were we moving during the two-week wait? What a waste of our last IVF round. Henri found me there, paralysed by pain, curled in a ball on the hard wooden floor. He helped me up and insisted I leave the house and go to the car. Henri does not drive, so it needed to be me, but I needed to rest first. He fed me tablets that did not touch the pain, then was forced to leave me alone to finish the house. I called my mother which triggered hysteria, when I heard her familiar voice, all warm and full of love, her voice that soothed me after the bullies hurt in school, her voice that whispered stories to me as a sleepy child, her voice that always made things less painful. Trying to take me down off the ceiling is no mean feat. She allowed me to bellow my anger into the phone and scream when the pain came in both my chest and my groin. My mother, my one constant, still mothering me at the grand old age of forty.

We needed to be gone. The house was no longer ours. The buyers are on their way to claim their new purchase.

There was much more to unpack than boxes when we got there.

Pregnant

Twenty minutes from Sherborne in another Dorset town, Andrew and Jane discovered they were once again pregnant. They had three children already, the oldest was just five, then a three-year-old, and a two-year-old. They were not only pregnant, but they were expecting twins, so they would go from three children to five. A big jump, they didn't know it yet, but it would become a leap too far for them to handle, already struggling with the children they had and their own addictions.

The Bit In Between

Recovery from the last failed IVF was just as painful as the previously failed IVF and the one before that, although this time, I had many more distractions. Travelling back to our old city to continue to work a couple of days a week, starting to hand over my clients from Lupilicious to various people who had worked for me.

In the apartment, the unpacking of endless brown boxes, as predicted, we needed the thickest underlay we could find laid to muffle the noise of Indian music wafting up through the floorboards with new carpet on top of that, sourcing a glazier to make bespoke glass for our windows so we could be warmer and to cancel out the noise from being sandwiched between two popular pubs, having our bathroom pulled out and replaced, painting wall after wall, an endless list of 'doing.'

I spent countless hours staring at the Abbey we lived in front of, a huge, strong, impenetrable, and remarkable stone structure, willing myself to stand just like it but failing. Failing again. I was aware my mental health had taken a huge battering over the last few years. Each day before I left my side of our bed, I wondered how I would survive the day; I just wanted to get back to the darkness. The cloak the darkness delivered gave me comfort, I could not be seen, I could draw the covers up over my head and sleep. I slept a great deal in those first months.

Selling our house had given us the repricve we craved from financial burden. We had a small nest egg for the first time since, well, since ever. When I approached the conversation I had been mulling over in my head for a few weeks now, I think Henri had been expecting it. I spoke very fast as if it would land better in amongst a jumble of words.

"I was chatting to my sister a few weeks ago, and she knows this really amazing doctor in fertility, he's written books, speaks on a world stage and he has a huge success rate. I was thinking we could pay for a round of IVF privately. I mean, I know it will cost, but we do have some cash now. What do you think? I want to. Why are you looking at me like that? What are you thinking? I really think we should give it another shot."

Silence.

"Yeah, no you're probably right, we can't really afford it, it would be all our money. Probably won't work. Same old. I am not sure anyone can help us." I blinked back, threatening tears and swallowed the huge lump in my throat that was making my voice sound thicker than normal.

Henri moved forward and bear hugged me. "Look, it's not that I don't want to go again, I just don't know how much more you can take. Let me take some time and think about it, ok?"

"I am forty years old. How much more time can we afford to take? Sorry, I don't mean to snap. It's been nearly eight years of trying and I am tired. Exhausted actually. My body is so tired of the medications. It is a lot. I mean, I reckon it can cope with another go. Just one more, but soon. Shall we? Can we?"

"I am not sure."

I press on. "I am, I am sure. Please, can I make an initial appointment?" Impatience is such a character flaw of mine.

"If you are sure you can cope? I can't witness you destroy yourself all over again, you feel broken still, it breaks my heart."

That is how we came to meet Dr Pole, an acclaimed fertility specialist otherwise known as 'the miracle baby maker.' He was based in a beautiful ornate surgery in a town not far from us with its own private car park, the kind where you drive in, and even the crunch of gravel feels grander than any of the hospitals we were used to. Walking in through huge, heavy doors with polished brass knobs and a shiny black paint finish, we were greeted by smiles from behind the reception desk. His waiting room was carpeted and warm with cushioned chairs to wait on. No peeling wall paint here. Tables of magazines like Vogue and Country Home and, of course, many copies of his books. We were offered tea or coffee to wait with. This is private care. The difference between what we had become accustomed to and what we were now sat in were worlds apart. Of course, this is what you pay for; the divide, the gap between the NHS and luxury, could not be any wider.

Dr Pole came to get us himself. A tall man dressed in suit trousers and a shirt with a tie, but there was a dishevelled, unironed look to him. His sleeves were rolled up and his hair floppy around his face and despite his age, he resembled a public school boy. He may have read my mind as he apologised for looking 'out of sorts' he was up in surgery at 6am and now it was 2pm and he had had no break in his day. I wanted to be sorry for him, but I did not have the space in my body for more emotion that morning. I was nervous and desperate. I wondered if he could see it.

Dr Pole was not like the other doctors we had met so far on this journey; he told us up front our chances of pregnancy were low just going by the file on our medical past and our ages. He needed to do some tests of his own and these would be done in his London clinics where the right cutting-edge equipment and labs available to him would be used. He wanted to know what the shape of my womb was, take new fresh internal scans to see for himself, and some more up-to-date bloodwork should be taken. We would get a letter with the appointment date soon.

"Are you sure this is what you want to do. We can do all this work and it still may not be the outcome you want. I need to be clear on that."

We nodded. Just like that he was showing us the door back to the waiting room. Twenty minutes and £250 quid later, we found a café, ordered coffee, and breathed out properly for what felt like the first time that day. I listened to Henri talking, being positive and light in conversation, but I felt heavy, my suitcase filling up again. Loss, failure, rejection, and desperation. I returned his smile and squeezed his hands, "I love you. Thank you for doing this again. I need one more spin of the wheel."

The letter detailing our appointments landed on the mat only five days later and only five days after that, I would be in Harley Street having all the tests Dr Pole had asked for done. We took the train. I felt a childlike excitement return; I felt safe in these new hands. I was more relaxed than I had been in months; it was a relief. We found a brasserie and had a simple lunch before finding our designated clinic, pressing on the shiny buzzer. We were shown upstairs, where I needed to fill my bladder to bursting point before, I could be scanned. I drank as much as I could from the glugging water cooler in the corner. It is no easy thing to fill your belly full of water, especially when it is so chilled. It is quite painful in truth.

A tall, slender female doctor called us into her office, a huge office that looked out on the busy street below. I wondered if those people hurrying to their next destination ever stopped to wonder what was happening in the buildings they rushed passed or if they were blissfully unaware that, in my case, this building housed such intimate procedures. I changed into a robe and lay on the couch. *Ok, let these new tests begin, just another couch and another pair of stirrups to hook my legs into. Shit, did I shave?* After a couple of hours of internal probes, waiting, scans, more waiting, and x-rays of my womb later, I was finally allowed to go to the loo. I dressed before six rounds of blood were taken from my veins. That was it, Dr Pole would be in touch.

Life just continued bumbling along whilst we waited for results.

I had two sessions left with one of my last remaining clients and then this business would be behind me. She was a busy working mother, often jet-setting around the world with her hugely successful mentoring business; her children were adopted, and she was open and vocal about it. She is all these things; glamorous, stunning, multi-linguistic, demanding, part of an elite group, unafraid, a straight talker, intimidating, and insecure. I liked her. She knew herself. I was her personal assistant, I cleaned up for her, did laundry, cooked food for supper, picked up her son from school, did homework with him, dog sat, did the shopping, sorted through whatever she needed me to, including her thoughts, I was both her part-time confidante and her hired help, and anything else that needed her attention.

The family home was old country chic, a vast home set in the Wiltshire countryside, full to bursting with very expensive and impressive items. Nothing was unaffordable for them; they could afford whatever they desired. It was fair to say she was incredibly disappointed about me leaving. She trusted me, I did a lot for her, but I was now leaving her to someone new. On my penultimate visit I was in her garden studio tidying around her whilst she was writing her first book. I remember her words very clearly, her words never beat around a bush getting to a point, they were always direct and if they touched a nerve, so be it. She put her pen down and looked up, taking her black thick rimmed glasses off and resting them on the desk as she leaned back in her antique chair, which creaked as she did so despite her small frame. "Loretta, have you thought this through?"

"Me leaving? Yes. Sorry, it's time for me to be in present in my life in one place."

"No, not that, although that is annoying, and I am not sure what I'll do yet. I mean, doing yet another tedious round of IVF. Don't you think it's a touch selfish?" She paused.

I stopped tidying as I could feel her eyes demanding I look at her, give her my full attention.

"Selfish?"

"Yes, if you could just get over yourself and your need to recreate your own genes, there are many children that are desperate for a family. Isn't that why you're doing IVF again? Genetics. It's selfish and quite vain, let's face it, all you want is a mini-me, someone who looks like you. If you ask me all this effort is pointless." She waved her hand dismissively around her head as if wafting away at an irritating invisible fly.

"Pointless?" I blinked back, tears threatening to fall and swallowed the lump in my throat. She had reached in and touched something inside me.

"Yes, all this medical drama for a child, you should get over yourself. Really. Anyway, think about it."

I could have been mad or should have been maybe, but I wasn't. Her way was pointed like that, and whilst I didn't ask for her input, I was used to it now. I knew she was trying to offer up some advice – you can't call it friendly or supportive advice but advice all the same. Was she right? Yes, she was, I did want our children to have my husband's kindness and mouth and my eyes. I wanted that. For them to look like us, to carry on our traits, our looks, our blood. If that made me selfish, well ok I accept that's what I am. We knew there were children waiting for homes, we had already committed to adopting at some point, but it is true we wanted our own first. Selfish. Yes. She was right.

She wasn't at home when I arrived for my last session with her. She left a note wishing me well.

Her words though, have always stayed with me.

I finished all my clients on the same day and good timing too, as the results from London were in. Before we could begin IVF number four, I needed an operation to remove a fallopian tube from my womb, and whilst Dr Pole was performing the surgery for me he would remove endometriosis as best he and his team could with his high-tech lasers. He had discovered that my womb was tilting at an awkward angle that could be an issue for transfer, I had a few fibroids (non-cancerous tumours in the womb) to be aware of and the results of my blood tests indicated nothing new or noteworthy. Operation date attached and will be performed at a London hospital with the pre-op in Dorchester at his clinic next week.

My womb was awkward. *What a surprise, I've been feeling awkward for a bloody lifetime. With this new discovery of a tilting womb, was he saying that the three IVF transfers I had previously had may have been successful if they had done a simple scan to find out the angle of my womb?* I rang the clinic as I needed to know to settle an incoming headache thinking about it. I could do nothing about it, but I needed to know. Shift the blame over a bit. Stop hating myself a little. Dr Pole took my call. "Possibly," is the best answer he could give me. "It's a possibility." I will cling to that.

Back off up to London, we went, making a weekend of it as my operation was on the Monday. We spent our time walking the streets in central London, eating food we couldn't get hold of down in Dorset like a decent Japanese, shopping for things we didn't need, visiting galleries, and plotting our future with an air of renewed hope. Autumn was all around us in nature as we wandered the streets of London. We kicked about the crispy orange and brown leaves fallen on the ground, the air smelled of smoke carried from the fires lit on the hearths of homes and pubs. A cosy slow weekend spent huddled together from the cold in the dark, early evenings.

Monday morning, we hailed a black cab to St Mary's Hospital. I had to check if it was, in fact, a hospital, as it just looked like a five-star hotel inside. I was shown to the second floor and my own room. Small but cosy. The hospital room, which looked out onto London's Hyde Park in the distance, was adorned with throws and cushions, a snug two-seater sofa in the corner, a large flat-screen TV on the wall with all the channels including Netflix, air conditioning, a small wardrobe, long mirror, and an array of complimentary soft drinks on a movable table that squeaked across the wooden floor as you moved it. The walls were painted in Farrow and Ball's Pale Hound. (Such a weird thing to know, but an old client once had me pouring over samples for her kitchen glow up.) It took a minute for it to feel real, then Henri reminded me none of this was free, we had, in fact, paid for this.

The friendly, chatty nurses prepped me for surgery and within two hours, I was wheeled into pre-op, talking to the anaesthetist and counting back from ten.

I woke in my room; I do not remember the post-operation room at all, but apparently, it took a while for me to come round. Opening my eyes, instinctively, I searched for Henri, his hand reached for mine. "Everything is done. It's good, now rest. I am here." The day shifted into night, I was in and out of sleep. When I woke at around ten in the evening, Henri had left for the hotel, the nurses had changed shifts, and the room was just about visible from a combination of the light coming into my room under the door from the corridor and the streetlamps shining in through the window. I was brought butter-soaked toast and a mug of steaming hot tea. Nothing tastes quite like this small meal after an operation.

I needed pain medication; I could feel a hot ball of rotating pain in my abdomen that was doing a good job at making my breath catch in my throat. All night, the pain came in and out in waves, as did my sleep and the demons in my nightmares. So grateful to see the morning light pour through the windows. I just wanted Henri and to go home. It wasn't long and Dr Pole was by my bedside checking me over for discharge. "Super job. All done. You are good to go home, but take it easy, you have just had big surgery."

Navigating a bustling Waterloo Station post-op was interesting. I felt like I needed a sign around me saying 'move away from this lady, parts of her are missing, she needs space.' I was not dealing with London's hustle of commuters and tourists well; my body was weak and delicate, my mind exhausted from the anaesthetic.

We were early for our train, so we rode the escalators to the balcony, ate comforting soup at Carluccios, looking down at the hordes of people all going their separate ways, lives to live, different journeys being taken.

Dr Pole that morning had told us that my defunct fallopian tube was an unusual dark grey in colour, so they were sending it off for testing to make sure it was not cancerous. *Good grief on top of all this do I have cancer too? Hello new level of anxiety, take a seat next to all the other active anxieties currently vying for my attention.* He had taken out what he described as "a ton of endometriosis which was 'no joke' to shift." The next step was to fully recover, then to attend a new appointment in Dorchester to create our IVF plan.

Private care was quick, it had an urgency to it. There were no queues, no other people to consider. Appointment. Plan. Invoice. Payment. Action. Next. A conveyor belt of efficiency with a smile.

The Knockout Round

Sitting in Dr Pole's office, I got a distinct feeling of déjà vu as we talked about our next and final round of IVF. I swiped surfacing old memories away as if they were an annoying wasp buzzing around my head, ready to sting at any moment. I did not want this to be like the other times; I did not want to even remember the other times right now. This was different (*wasn't it?),* so I shoved the feeling away as far as my mind could hurl it. I forced a smile as my attention came back to listening to new plans being made and the processes to follow. This IVF had started to take shape, except it was almost an identical plan to the last three attempts ... déjà vu crept back in, laughing in my face.

The medication arrived swiftly. I packed it into a cleared space in the fridge for one final time. Last chance saloon.

Around the two-week mark into the course of injecting, we had an appointment to separately see a medium and tarot card reader. Some people doing IVF get acupuncture, some try reflexology, others pray, and some even just trust the process. We went 'woo woo'. Henri was sold less on this route than I was. I grew up with a mother that loved to see a tarot card reader and each time she went, there was something quite uplifted in her attitude when she returned.

I have had my own run in with the spiritual world, so I, like my mother, have a sort of blind faith in these psychic readers.

....

Saturday afternoon inside the big City Hall building, two years before I met Henri and having just moved to the area, a Psychic Fair was in full swing. I decided, with nothing else to do and no friends made yet, that I would go in and have a wander round. I passed stalls selling crystals and dream catchers, healing and massages happening behind screens, people selling past life regression sessions, and rows of tarot card readers lined up around the edges of the huge room that is usually reserved for theatre or live music. I spotted a Reiki taster session in the middle of the room, £5 for ten minutes. Having never tried it, let's see what it's like. I sat on an old-school wooden chair, the Reiki master told me to relax, to close my eyes, and enjoy. I was tired that day, moving down from Berkshire had been a big decision and I hadn't really settled into my new life yet. I remember thinking of nothing, just enjoying being able to close my eyes with the sounds of the people and treatments around me playing in my ears. I was free, free as a bird, almost literally, I seemed to be floating at ceiling height of this vast room looking down at the fair going on beneath me. I recognised a girl that I had met that week at my new workplace at one of the jewellery stalls arguing with her boyfriend. I watched all the tarot card readers, there must have been around thirty and from my bird's eye view I chose to go and see a woman wearing a red jacket sat at her table smiling at her customer as she looked heavenward. She had a really colourful shimmer to her, I believe it was her aura, whatever it was I liked it. I floated around happily watching from my newly acquired position. Without warning I felt a pain hit my chest. Was someone throwing stones at me? I started to fall from the ceiling. Falling from this height wasn't going to end well. With a jolt I opened my eyes to searing pain in both my feet. I seem to have drawn a crowd of people around me; I had not fallen to the ground in a heap but still sat on the wooden chair blinking at the bright lights in the room. To my left concerned on-site paramedics and to my right quite the distraught reiki master. The pain in my feet was where the heavier of the paramedics and the reiki master had jumped on my feet in unison in a last attempt to wake me from my reverie. They had apparently tried jabbing fingers into my chest. Not stones, pokey fingers, the result of which were blossoming bruises. I had been out for around thirty minutes apparently. After lots of fuss and bother, I ended up comforting a very distraught reiki healer, assuring him I was, in fact, okay and that I wasn't a witch. *Okay not the witch bit, but what was that that happened?*

Dazed a little, my feet still recovering, I limped over to the woman in red. When I sat down, I told her what had just happened with the reiki master (who I could see packing up his pitch, still looking perplexed) and she laughed, throwing her head back before she told me she had looked up when she was with her last customer as she thought she was being watched from above by a lingering presence. She was quite relieved I wasn't a gatecrashing spirit. She read my cards with absolute clarity. I was shit out of luck on the love front for a few years still when two men would come into my life at once but rest assured, I would choose the right one. Sure enough, around two years later, there were two men, best friends but Henri was my choice.

....

I was curious once more. I say curious, but what I wished for from this medium was to tell me that this last IVF round would work, that we would be pregnant, let's be honest, that is all I wanted to hear.

We once tried the acupuncture route before the second IVF, I had my appointment with a Chinese acupuncturist who had a very good reputation in the area, and he asked me a variety of questions, including when the round was starting. I replied, six weeks. He concluded that it wouldn't work for me because I was too fat, and six weeks was no time to lose weight and start the course of acupuncture. His exact words were 'too fat to conceive.' I almost ran from his surgery in shame.

I knocked on our medium's big, old heavy set wooden door first, Henri waited in the café across the street. Linda showed me to her shed at the end of her garden. It was perhaps what you would expect from a medium's room with its wicker furniture and plump cushions, crystals, burning incense, and angel statues, the vibe was warm and cosy. Easy to settle into. Linda resembled Ma Larkin from the book *The Darling Buds of May* that I'd read as a child. She was chubby and cheerful, with pure love in her soul, I just wanted her to pull me into a hug. My session was peppered with facts I already knew, which is a good sign when someone does not know you from any other person walking down a busy high street. She told me plenty, but nothing I wanted to hear. Something about me working in a jewellery shop which made no sense at all. I had never once been interested in making jewellery or selling it, I just loved wearing it. I came away disappointed. I asked her right at the end, before I said goodbye, what was the outcome of this IVF and she said she couldn't tell me that or it would skew the path. *O for goodness' sake. What was the point?*

I stomped across the road the way a small child would if they had been told no to sweets in the supermarket. I opened the café door with force fueled by my frustration, making people turn in their seats to see who was bringing in the cold autumnal breeze as the little bell rang out above the door announcing my arrival at the same time. Soothed almost instantly by the smell of coffee and toast. Hungry. I needed breakfast. Clearly hunger has kicked in. Henri quickly kissed me, smiled, and left for his session. We had booked separately for the same day, so Linda had no idea Henri and I even knew each other let alone were a married couple. Henri went so far as to take his ring off to throw her off the scent. We had factored in that if she was the real deal, she would know no matter what we did.

After over an hour and a half and three cups of coffee, that impatient part of me, which is probably 70% of me at most of any given time, felt Henri had been gone for too long and I mulled over knocking on her door to find out what was keeping him there. Just at that point, he walked through the door. A waitress greeted him a welcome back and would he like another coffee? He sat. I stared at him.

"Well, come on. Anything?"

Grinning, he said, "It's BOGOF. My grandad Lenny was there, he told me, it's BOGOF. Also, it must be legit cause he appeared to Linda holding a fallopian tube. I mean, that is a bit weird. How would she know that! Your fallopian tube is with my grandad, which incidentally is a sentence I never thought I would say. So, yeah, BOGOF."

"What the hell is BOGOF?"

"Buy one get one free. So, like twins, I guess."

"OMG we are going to have twins?"

"Looks that way if we believe the 'woo woo'!"

All my disappointment was abandoned. I have never felt so elated, so overjoyed. Filled full of hope for the first time since IVF number one.

I knew it, this was different. Surely now was our time.

Scan day arrived and we were once again sent home as the eggs were not growing as they should be, and of course, new medication arrived to help with that. Ten extra days added to the cycle. It didn't matter, though, as I was so buoyed by Henri's session with Linda. I was convinced twins were about to be unconventionally conceived.

Around the same time, we were planning to start a new barbershop business in a shop we had looked at on the high street. We had searched our local high street and waited for the right empty premises to come up. Most were too small, and one situated right next door to another barbershop, so opening there would mean inviting trouble in from the off. The premises that had recently become available, situated in the middle of the high street, big enough for a barbershop with up to four cutting chairs with rooms upstairs we could rent out, not only that, it had bags of charm and character. We arranged a viewing. We fell in love with the shop and its high ceilings, huge, old, lead windows, and quirky small entrance door. It needed work; some of the carpet had been lifted in one corner of the room; on inspection, we could see beneath a beautiful wooden floor waiting to be uncovered. There was no boiler, which didn't alarm us given that our flat didn't have any heating either. The business inside it, before it emptied out, was a jewellery business and had closed due to lack of trade. Although the rumours were its demise could have also been to do the frosty reception when entering the shop, I am not talking about the lack of heating.

A jewellery shop, Linda had predicted something around jewellery, and I had laughed it off. Chatting later to my mother about the premises, she reminded me it was also where my grandfather used to buy his tobacco for his pipe-smoking habit in the 1980s when he and my grandmother came up from Devon to live with us in the annexe attached to my childhood home. Just knowing he had been in there, walked those floorboards, combined with Linda's prophecy was comfort enough for me to feel this location was meant to be for us. Henri's daily commute needed to come to an end as it was tiring travelling an hour each way every day and working the long ten-hour days. Plus, with our IVF round ramping up and the real possibility of becoming a family of five (four humans and a furry woof), our first barbershop started to look for a manager or, more preferably, a buyer.

IVF injections, planning, employing, commuting. It all rumbled on. Our new normal, albeit far from actual normality, but to us, it had become the humdrum. Day in, day out. We injected, Henri commuted, I made our flat into a home, completed admin and planning for the new shop, Henri came home. We flumped on the sofa most nights, Henri exhausted from work, me exhausted from all the meds.

The days rolled by and most of those, I was sat on the floor of what would become the nursery just staring at the walls as they came alive with my daydreams of what life would look like, how I would nurse them through the night, sing lullabies, change nappies, read books, and watch them sleeping. I planned yellow, not the garish in-your-face yellow but a pale subtle yellow. Non-gender specific. I searched for children's wall stickers; I fancied something fun like a circus theme. All the fun of the fair, well something like that, not so strange that I had chosen that theme with my feeling that the whole IVF journey resembled the chaos of a circus. The nursery was sandwiched in between our room and the sitting room in our strangely laid out multi-floored apartment. Digby had already taken up residence outside their door as a preferred sleeping spot. Their own fluffy guard dog.

Egg collection day arrived, and once again, I would be going under general anaesthetic for them to carefully remove the eggs in my ovaries that I had laboriously grown with the assistance of the injections. Our great friend Emma drove us to Dorchester very early in the morning in her little Fiat. As they chatted breezily in the front of the car, I watched the fields rush by and my eye wandered into the distance to where the blue sky met the green horizon of rolling Dorset countryside. I remember not thinking very much, more pushing back the fear and anxiety that this would end the same way as all the other rounds as thoughts tried to sneak in through any means possible. My heart skipped beats, so I steadied it. My lungs felt short of air, so I purposely took big, long, deep breaths, my brain tried to present negativity, my stomach flipping somersaults, so I held it tight.

Back under and out of general anaesthetic within twenty minutes, a nurse was bringing me round from what always feels like hours and hours of sleep. It is so hard to come round from that kind of sedation. Groggily, I asked her, "Did they get enough?" She didn't reply, had I said it in my head? "The eggs, did they get good ones?"

"O, yes, it's all fine." Then my mind quickly wondered how Henri got on in his little room with a stack of dog-eared magazines and his imagination.

Emma scooped us up from the hospital and drove us home. She happily chatted all the way and I drifted off to the sound of her voice. I love her vocal tones, I used to fall asleep listening to her stories when we were sharing a room at boarding school. It has a rich warmth to it, marshmallows after the heat of roasting them on an open fire. She is a safe place.

The next day, we eagerly awaited news on our embryos. The phone not out of my sweaty palm for more than a minute until it rang with news. All had gone well overnight; two embryos had died off, but three were looking strong. The transfer was to happen the next day at 10am.

We were at the hospital at 9am and told to go home until midday to give the embryos a few hours more. One more embryo had died that morning. That meant none to freeze again. It's ok, it's all going to be ok.

Coffee and toast were ordered in a nearby urban-style coffeehouse and whilst the coffee started to work its dark magic, making me more alert, my appetite had deserted me. Henri too, it would seem, judging by his still full plate. He held my hands. "No matter what happens, I love you. We are doing this together. You carry the embryos, and I will carry you." Tears sprung to the corners of my eyes, and I looked at him through the watery blur, blinking to allow the tears to flow down my face. For the first time this round I voiced my deep fear, "What if this doesn't work? What do we do?"

"If it doesn't, we take a breath, and decide what the next step is together."

"I don't think I can do this again. My body feels wrecked and bloated…" Henri cut in. "Stop projecting, let's do this one step at a time. This round is not over."

It's not over. I stood up filled with love and bolstered by Henri's support, ready for transfer number four.

IVF round four lasted thirteen days. We nearly made it. The embryos gave up on day thirteen. Always was my unlucky number.

The Fog of Grief

To unpick the last five years or so was nothing short of hard work. I had to look inward for the answers and that meant starting back at my childhood, my new therapist explained. To find forgiveness, to forgive myself, I needed to delve deep to uncover what was in the dark. A little like mining for gold nuggets, it was mostly darkness, but coming across a piece of gold felt special; it sparkled. Those sparkles shed light on the pathway out of the shadows.

Straight after the fourth failed IVF, two things happened that I wasn't expecting. The first thing was that I felt relief. It was over. We were not trying again. Done. Our doctor had said that really the chances were so low now; a forty-year-old woman with endometriosis, adenomyosis, fibroids and endometrioma. We could try the surrogate route or maybe fly out to Greece, as the track record there for IVF is better than in the UK. I didn't bother to ask why it wasn't so good right here from this office with all the thousands of pounds we had spent with him. I was tired. I felt old. My mind felt muddy, nothing was quite clear, focus was temporarily disabled, joy, laughter along with it. Numbness consumed my whole self, body, and mind. Henri made the decision in the end, and I have never been more grateful to him. He read me; he knew. His journey and his dream too, crushed. We needed to heal. There were no next steps.

The second thing was an overwhelming feeling of hatred. I truly hated myself. My body was a complete failure and it had been left further ravaged by the medications, treatments, and injecting. It was a bloated, puffy version of me. It had been a pin cushion, subjected to endless intrusive operations, filled to the brim with drugs and steroids. It had been the victim of doctors' poking, prodding, it had had parts removed or lasered off, it had tried and failed to grow babies, it was soaked in medical ailments, and it had on numerous occasions been called too fat by professionals and myself. I had bullied my own body. My mind too was weak. Why had I not been stronger? My mental health throughout had taken a beating and now it was only capable of going through the daily motions. My face smiled but it lied. I was a fake, a fraud, I was anything but the smiling front I presented to the world.

Digby and I would walk. A lot. Long isolated walks. Ask me what I was thinking about in those walks I won't be able to tell you. It's like I emptied my mind into the atmosphere, and it had become just an empty vessel capable of the very basic actions. No thoughts. That is why I took so much time walking, doing that activity wiped it all for a moment in time, I gave it all up to the nature around me to disperse it as it saw fit. The guilt, the blame, and the shame. Silence in my head, just my eyes resting on the beauty of nature surrounding me, keeping me calm, stable. This stillness amongst nature knew instinctively how to grieve and be reborn is where my love (and hate) relationship started with jogging. I found the further I jogged, the longer the pressure in my head was released. Nothing but one foot in front of the other and some old school, house music blasting in my ears, drowning out any thoughts that remained.

It wasn't enough though. Half an hour afterwards, the endorphins had worn off and I was back to feeling heavy in my limbs and my thoughts. I talked and cried a great deal with Henri, and I only felt safe wrapped in his arms like I may have fallen apart if he was not nearby. I became needy, like a child would in crisis.

In stark contrast to the exercise I was doing, I ate. Stuffing my face with junk, momentary happiness, the food would bury the emotions I didn't want to face, stuffing down anything negative.

Henri tried to talk to me about the possibilities of adoption, at that point, I was pulverised to a sort of nothingness. I wasn't meant to be a mother and the universe was telling me so. Then I would cry more about what our children would have looked like, how they would have been and that I was a faulty woman. I cried at everything, the adverts for the abused donkeys carrying water in third world countries on the TV, someone else's trauma when their dog accidentally jumped off a cliff, my grandfather's death and how much I still missed him fifteen years later, the babies we didn't get to hold in our arms.

One warm summer's evening on a gentle meander into the fields, the sun's last golden rays were soaking into our skin, the birds were still chirping, but it had quietened from this morning when the crickets and bees were busy creating and alongside that, summer hum buzzing around as the day heats up, was when Henri very gently asked me if I thought I was depressed. It stopped me in my tracks. I stared at him and started to cry. "Do you think I am?"

"Yes. I do." He took my hands. "Depression is not your failure. It is brought about from our situation. I think we need to find you some help. Someone for you to talk to. Someone that is just for you."

"How can we afford it? I mean, we spent the money we had on bloody useless IVF." I could feel the anger rising again.

"We will find a way. I need you to find your joy again. I miss you."

Therapy. Ok. Ok. Don't really messed up people do therapy?

"Babe, really screwed up, people have therapy. Am I really that messed up?"

"You are in a muddle and not able to see your self-worth, you hate yourself. That is not normal. You punish yourself. I think you are full of grief and that needs to come out, like it needs to be purged from you. I love you, but it's not enough. So yeah, a bit messed up!" He gave me a squeeze.

For the first time in what feels like forever, I laughed. He had voiced it, exactly what I had been thinking. Messed up.

Depressed. Low. He is right, I cannot continue to live under a dark cloud, in the shadows. I do need help.

When I stop laughing, I sob with relief into his chest. I don't need to shrivel up and quietly live a life of unfeeling and sadness, I can fix myself, with help. I can maybe find a way out of the shadows. I took Henri's hand and watched Digby running after a butterfly in the field, calmness returning to my body.

"Do you think I can heal enough so we can start the adoption process?"

Henri winked, "I was hoping you were going to say that, but you have to come first!"

It took me a while to find a therapist because it had to be someone that I felt comfortable with in conversation, someone whose voice sounded kind but wise. I finally spoke to a woman over the phone whose voice was soft and calm, as opposed to clipped and terse. She didn't interrupt me when I was making my long-winded enquiry; she gave me space to talk, but she had no room for new clients. After speaking to four other therapists in the area, I phoned her to tell her I would wait. In no more than three weeks, a space came available, and I booked my first session.

On the day of my first session, I was nervous. I had no idea what to expect. Her house was an old residence tucked away down a single hidden track. I walked up her uneven red brick garden path with thirsty summer flowers falling on top of it from each side. I stopped at the red brick porch and tucked in between the faded yellow front door and its frame was a note addressed to me.

> 'Come on in and shut the door. Head down the corridor through the connecting door and straight up both sets of stairs. At the top go up the three steeper steps, turn left and come down the next corridor. I will hear you and greet you but please do not use the

knocker on the front door in case I am in session still.
Pru'

As I stepped inside, I was greeted with a smell, a combination of a shepherd's pie cooking in the oven and damp. The walls in the hallway were a dirty cream that needed a fresh lick of paint. It was dark and cool, especially coming in from the bright, warm sunshine outside. I passed so many closed doors as I headed up the corridor to the stairs. Each footstep creaked with every step I took; it was so quiet that I felt like I was trespassing. Once I got to the top of the three steeper steps taking me up to another floor, a door opened and out walked Pru. She smiled warmly and gave me a cheery welcome.

"Hello Loretta, come in, come in."

Therapy, My New Best Friend

My new therapist was not dressed as I had imagined her to be from our initial phone call. Her soft, unhurried tones had suggested a neutral person in my mind's eye, a woman who wore long skirts and colours to match that voice. Pru was not this person; she was probably in her late fifties, maybe early sixties, and wore plenty of bright colours. Her tights were purple, her skirt just above the knee, a white shirt poking out under a soft but thin, mustard V-neck jumper. Not a scrap of makeup; her skin was supple and flawless. Her eyes bright and her hair short and grey in tights curls. I quickly realised that I had placed her in a box labelled 'clever but no zest for life' in my head, like I would for an accountant, or tax person and this was the first of my mistakes with Pru. Clever yes, boring and drab she was not.

I was invited to sit in a chair inside the bay window. As I walked to the chair, I looked out the window into her big overgrown beautifully untidy garden that reminded me of an orchestra prepping for a big night ahead. It struck me that the garden was alive, living its life to its full potential. I wondered if I would soon be transformed like that garden. So many variants of green from thriving plants and trees, pops of colour from an assortment of flowers which made me think of Pru's dress sense. From this window, I could see butterflies and bees in what looked to me like a small slice of heaven. I turned back into the room and sat down. To my left was a sofa and to my right, a table with a box of tissues on it. As I swept the room, I noticed books, so many books which made me smile, I liked a room with books in it. As my eyes came to rest on her she was smiling at me.

"Let me tell you how these sessions work. You talk and I listen. I will give challenge and guide you deeper allowing you to work your way through your pain so you can manage it and get on top of it. OK? Let's begin."

"Ok." I waited and she smiled. I felt that familiar awkwardness seeping in, almost like I was in fact still trespassing on the stairs and I briefly acknowledged that I felt that way a lot. "What shall I say? What do you need from me?"

"I don't need anything from you." She paused and I must have looked like I'd been caught out somewhere I shouldn't be. "Ok let's start by you telling me why you are here, and we will go from there."

Deep breath. Please do not cry. "Well, I don't really know, but I do know that I feel sort of broken. Non-operational. Defunct."

Silence, so I filled it.

"I feel messy in my head, the way a ball of wool looks after a kitten has played with it for a while. I can't untangle it. I have failed again and again. My body has betrayed me. IVF failed us and now I need help to get past it. My family doesn't want to talk to me about it. It feels like they don't care, I don't think it is true, but no one wants to approach me about it. I am new to this town and barely have any friends. Well, none actually. I just don't see the point of anything anymore. Nothing makes sense." Tears had sprung, a golf ball-sized lump in my throat was restricting my voice making me sound a lot higher pitched than normal, bordering on hysteria.

"Please take a tissue." I shook my head preferring instead to use my sleeve the way a child would. I felt like a child. I felt small in that chair.

"What do you mean, 'again'. You failed again, and again?"

"All my life, I seem to scrape by leaving a trail of destruction behind me. Failure upon failure. I don't mean to, but I do tend to get myself in impossible situations. No one else I know seems to make the mistakes I make. Maybe it would just be a huge mistake to be a mother. That's why I can't get pregnant."

"Loretta, life does not work that way. There's a lot to unpack here and to do this we need to go backwards. Right back to your childhood before we could answer your more immediate questions. Tell me about your childhood; your mother and father, siblings. What was it like growing up being you?"

Just like that, I was transported back to being four years old, so now I didn't just feel like a child in that chair, but I was seeing my childhood laid out in front of me. Where to begin. "My earliest memory really, I suppose, is living above my parents' restaurant before we moved to the big house and whilst they were working downstairs, I spoke into a little speaker hooked up on the skirting board outside my room if I needed something. The little speaker's wire ran all the way down to my father's kitchen downstairs. Both my parents worked the evenings, so my sister and I were left unattended. They could hear us and talk to us, but we were left alone. That little tinny speaker got me into trouble. I remember having a friend over to stay and we were playing dress up instead of sleeping and she had my new nurse's outfit on, and I wanted it back, I said, 'give it bloody back'. I heard my name shouted from the floor where the speaker was plugged in, followed by footsteps stamping up the stairs. My mother burst into the room and reprimanded me for swearing. She pulled me to the bathroom and literally washed my mouth out with a bar of soap. I won't ever forget it. The shame and embarrassment in front of my friend. Then there was the time that we got a golden Labrador puppy, Susie, and she was left in the bathroom when they went down to work. I was a child excited by this furry cute bundle so, I crept as quietly as I could to go in and be with her as she was whimpering and the speaker roared, 'go back to bed' making me jump out of my skin. I hated that speaker. Mostly because it was a snitch but mainly because it replaced my parents six nights a week."

Therapy had started and it was nothing like I had imagined it would be. No bed to lie on, no notes being taken, no glasses balanced on a therapist's nose. It was colourful, just how life should be.

Injecting Colour Not Meds

Every week, on the same day at the same time, I landed in Pru's colourful room full of books, we quickly identified I needed two sessions a week to start with. This room is where I spilt it all, my safe space. I opened the cracks in my life wider, turning them into gaping holes, bravely allowing the pain to flow in and out. I didn't realise the extent of damage that had been done over my whole life leading up to these moments inside this pale-yellow room with a view of passing seasons.

I talked about my family and my childhood, school, friendships, the appalling men that had drifted in and out of my life, my husband, the babies that never came. I talked about me and as I talked, I did not recognise huge parts of myself. I really have not been living, more existing and the amount of people pleasing I had been doing made me so mad. I got angry. Why have I spent a good majority of my life living for other people's recognition? How does a person get to that place?

For a long while, I became worse, I was completely and utterly shattered, an empty shell of the person I once was. The person I knew to be me, was taken down bit by bit, the pieces of me at my feet. Together Pru and I were pulling all of myself off the bones to sift through the meaty debris before slowly and carefully putting back the pieces that were the essence of me. The other pieces of me, the pieces that hurt, made me want to crawl inside the human-sized shell we broke open more, faced the trauma of them then I mentally locked them in a box, not to forget but because they were now dealt with, less poison more learnt lessons. No longer did I need to carry that load around with me. I had thrown away that tatty old suitcase.

Life was changing. I was changing. Everything was becoming more fluid, like a blockage slowly being removed.

After each session I took to going for a run as soon as the hour had finished. Running gave me space and clarity. I would run out into the woods and other faraway places; nothing would be in my head except the words of the music blaring out from my headphones. Sometimes the music became me, it carried me away and emotions would build into my chest making me so breathless I would have to stop and gulp in some air. As I doubled over breathing hard, the tears would come and the grief would spill from my eyes, wailing from my lungs, my mind awash with images of loss. Allowing myself to feel all the pain was healing me.

The childhood I held in my mind's eye was not the childhood I lived. The aesthetics were all real but the life I had lived was different to the stories I used to regale so often about my early years. I spent a lot of time alone as my parents' worked evenings. They worked so hard. If I ever questioned why we were left so alone, the answer was always that it was all for my sister and I, our future. I learned to understand that whilst I went to a private school, wearing a uniform of kilt, shirt, tie, and a boater, and had access to all the privileges that came with that school, I would have preferred to have attended a state school and see more of my parents, have family time. Instead of the brand-new car on the drive gifted to me when I was seventeen years old, I would have preferred an old banger to have been with my parents more. Instead of the house with the beautiful garden, tennis court, double garage, and fields, I would have preferred to live on a normal street with neighbours that you would say good morning to you every day and seen my parents more. I had grown up lonely and unparented. I had to learn for myself. My parents loved me hard, but they valued creating money for our future as a necessity over nurturing us. I had all I needed, except the connection I craved for.

When my grandparents came to live with us, Gran was poorly diagnosed with Alzheimers and Parkinsons, it had become safer for them to live with us. My grandfather, who I had always adored became my hero in those years. I clung on to him so tightly, I was his shadow, in return, I was enveloped with love. Our bond was set beforehand but in all the years we lived together it was cemented, I needed him, and he saw that but, in some way, he needed me too. He parented me and taught me so much about living, his values are still some of the values I live by today. So, of course, when he died it hit me as if I had been run over by a truck. I was knocked off my feet, I did not understand it at the time as I was so consumed with sadness, that I wasn't meant to just carry on, I was meant to stop and grieve. I didn't grieve him until Pru handed me the key to unlock myself, then I had no choice but to see that all those years without him for what they were; I was misfiring, running on empty, lonely again. I put myself in those shitty situations to punish myself because it was easier to feel pissed off than grieve for him and acknowledge his death and my loss.

Therapy was my lifeline whilst I was in it. I uncovered parts of me I had deliberately hidden, discovered who I was, peeled back the layers of protection as you would a fleece on a seedling plant so it can soak in the sunshine and grow. I am not sure where I would be without having had gone through it.

One year in and our sessions were down to one a week, the crying had become less of a centrepiece as I started to understand why I had come to be the person I was when I first walked into Pru's yellow room. I understood it but I was still angry at it. Pru said until I got a handle on that I still had work to do.

"Initially, I came because I wanted to help myself through the IVF grief. Is it not time we got to it; we have not touched upon that yet, not even close."

"We have not. For us to start that avenue, you needed to know who you were, who you can be. There would have been no way you could heal your IVF grief when you were grieving for so many other parts of your life. There were no endings because you couldn't bear to close them. You had no support to do that. Look how far we've come, the road has been rocky and uphill and you have bravely taken each part and confronted it, torn it down and remoulded it into something you understand, something more manageable. You are stronger now. It is now that you can tackle the enormity of your baby losses."

"Baby losses?"

"Mmhmm. Loss. Let's talk about the babies you have lost."

Right there in the safety of the little yellow room, I understood. All that I am is not why I am not a mother. In fact, it is why I should be a mother. I have come through the other side of a mountain of trauma. In my forty-odd years, I have faced a childhood that dealt with working parents not present to be with me, stood by and helplessly watched my grandparents decline in health, been bullied in school, friendships that time and again became toxic, my father not speaking to me for three years as I chose to be in London over the family business, nearly losing my father in a near-fatal car accident, the isolation of living in London, my parents divorcing, raped by a now shamed celebrity, drug use, and lost a few years of my life to it, men controlling me for their own gains, boyfriends that left destruction in my life, losing my precious connection with my sister for a while, gaining weight, loneliness, so much loneliness. Eight long years trying for a family of my own.

I was now in a place where I had spent a year grieving it all, accepting it all. The noose was loosening from around my neck. The heaviness in my limbs is becoming lighter.

My therapy process also celebrated the good stuff too, Pru and I prioritised it. Being the first person in my family to get a degree, meeting Henri, Digby, marrying Henri, reconnection with my sister, moving back to be near family, running my first 5km race, setting up successful businesses, working through the issues with my father and enjoying him as I did when I was a small child. I survived against the odds. Acknowledging that I am a person of worth, that I am clever and full of love to give. That I am deserving of a good life.

Only strong women need apply. I am one of them. I was ready to face the last eight years and simultaneously Henri and I were ready to start the adoption process. Ready to let colour back in, start laughing and living life again.

Part Three
The Adoption Years

Welcome To Social Services

Back on the family-making start line. On your marks, get set, go!

We quickly learnt that the process to adopt a child is nothing like just popping in an application form, having a few chats, and being allocated a child. I didn't think it would be that easy of course, but I thought there would be some guidance and support, at the very least from a Google search, a 'how to' for the first steps into the world of adoption. I know some people had adopted abroad some years ago via the church and all you needed back then was a wad of cash and a promise. So, our search on Google turned up nothing except making it plain to see that we needed to dig quite a lot deeper.

Before IVF, when we had tried to climb aboard the adoption train, it was through the local council services, so we reluctantly started back there again. I wanted to adopt from abroad, so many orphanages were full to bursting in countries less wealthy than the UK, but it turns out it all started with local council approval. To adopt abroad you need to have gone through the application procedure via the council. Anything council-related feels a bit of a laborious route to a family. I said that to Henri, and he laughed "What did you expect, an Angelina Jolie and Brad Pitt route to adoption?" Well, no, just something less beige.

We called the County Council and were directed to the social services department, where a cranky older lady picked up the phone. The call went a little like this:

Papers were rustling, something fell on the floor, an audible groan. "Social Services."

"O hello!" (I put on my very chirpy, happy, you will absolutely love us, voice) "We are looking to start the adoption process."

Silence.

"Erm, am I in the right place?"

"Hmm? Ok, yes you are." Something falls to the floor, "Bugger, ooo sorry, one of those days, right, long old road adoption."

"Well, yes. I mean we have been ther..."

"Right, I'll stop you there, you need to come to an information evening. Give me your email address and I'll send over our address and the timings, all the gumpf you need. Email back to say if you're coming."

That was it. In true British fashion, in keeping with doctor receptionists, hospital receptionists, school receptionists, in fact, any receptionist I have ever been in contact with the conversation was short and not so sweet, bordering rude.

The email arrived two days later. The contents of which contained a date, time, and an address with the sign off 'let us know if you are attending.' No gumpf included. I emailed back to say we were attending and jotted down our names. I did not get a reply and somehow, I was not shocked.

We drove thirty minutes to an information session we weren't quite sure we were booked onto and arrived in the car park, which sat in front of a beautifully old grey brick but shabby-looking building, it could have once been a manor house. We parked and sat in silence watching people in the same situation as our own walking in. Not a room full of pregnant couples but couples just like us. Climbing out of our car, smoothing down our clothes, holding hands to support one another, we walked to the entrance. Unlike IVF, this process involved us both in equal parts and I found a strange comfort in that, this route, we were both responsible for the outcome.

It was dark and musty inside, the walls paneled with dark wood, on the right of the entrance hall a tiny window sat at shoulder height with glass filling its hole. The glass window slid open with a clunk, indicating the glass had found it couldn't be pushed any further, and an invisible receptionist barked 'Yes?' through the hole. 'It's that building,' she gestured with her hand popping up into the glassless hole back out to the car park. On the side of the building was a modern building, not unlike a mobile classroom from the seventies. No one noticed us as we walked in, so we started to walk towards the other side of the room, where we spied two free seats. The layout was similar, in fact, to a classroom with the tables pushed into a U shape, we sat on blue plastic chairs that scraped the floor as we pulled them out, we sat down and faced the front where a woman had her back to us and was fussing and grunting over an overhead projector.

The three ladies that seemed to be overseeing the meeting all having had a go at making the technology work, one at a computer offering instructions from a website, another on her phone, before the woman gave up on the overhead projector with plenty of audible sighing and turned into the room, towards us, her audience. The woman sat in the middle, clearly still frustrated the overhead projector did not work, said, "Right we had better get started as it's nearly time for dinner." They introduced themselves and sat down, one dropped her entire file on the floor in the process of taking a seat, she groaned and fell to her knees in amongst her self-imposed debris to scoop up all the papery mess. A tiny younger woman was croaked at, a sharp order to hand out information sheets to each of us and the croaker sat like the Queen frog on a lily pad, waiting for her team to come back to her.

The hour whizzed by. We had so much information thrown at us so quickly that I suspected dinner was, in fact, very nearly ready, bordering on ruined. We learnt that many people in that room won't bother coming back, some will make it past the home visits before giving up, and the majority of us will be gone during the application process. Nothing like a good dose of positivity at the start line of our new chapter.

Apparently, it took a certain type of person to adopt but it was not so apparent who that type of person was.

There would be days of training that we had to attend, if we could not go due to prior commitments, our application would be terminated. Mandatory attendance. The application form was allegedly epic in its volume, we needed to expect it to take between three to six months to complete. Then there was the Panel Board to get through as well. If we were still interested in moving forward, we needed to be allocated a social worker, so we needed to email them to give confirmation that we were giving the green light to go ahead. She wrapped up the session with, "Right, let's get home for some dinner. Are there any questions?" No one dared ask her anything as dinner seemed to be hanging in the balance.

We waited. Patiently. We did not want to rock the boat by asking why our social worker had not yet been allocated, we couldn't possibly appear to be impatient parents in waiting. By week three of waiting, though, I summoned the courage and my cheeriest voice to call the receptionist again.

"Good morning! Wondering if I can speak to the adoption department."

"Uh huh, I need to know why before I can put you through."

"We are waiting on our social worker allocation, and we have not heard back yet. It's been a little while, so I thought I'd give you a ring."

"Right then, hang on." To my surprise she popped us through to the department, and a different lady picked up the phone.

"Adoption team."

"Hi, we attended the last information session you ran, and we are waiting for a social worker allocation so we can get started. Please. Thank you."

"Ok. Hmm. Right. I need to find your paperwork. O damn it. Sorry! I just dropped some files. What are your names?" I had a sneaking suspicion this was the lady that had dropped her files before and scattered her organisation all over the floor.

"Loretta and Henri Lupi-Lawrence."

"Hmmmm. Right. Let me see. Did you come to an information evening? I don't see your names anywhere."

"Yes, yes we definitely came along." My voice, I noticed, had gone up a few octaves.

"Hmmmm. Let's say you have then. Did you email in your interest afterwards?"

"O yes straight away, we would really like to get started."

"Yes, I hear you it's a very long process you do understand that. Right Ok. O I just found your email. Don't know how I missed that. Whoopsie. Ok well the team are fully allocated at the moment. I'm just going to pop you on hold. Two secs."

Without realising, I start to pace the living room and I seem to be cleaning surfaces with my sleeve. I should just get a duster, but if I go into the kitchen, I may lose reception, so I will stay where I am anxiously cleaning objects and shelving with my black long sleeved top whilst I wait.

Nearly ten minutes later, "Hmmm hello? Right then. Are you still there? As I thought the team is fully booked up with potential adoptees and cases on their desks, so I have allocated you Doreen for the moment. How's next Wednesday at ten o'clock, it's the only slot she has got for a while? I think I can see your address from the email. Yes, got it."

Air punch, little dance on the spot. "Absolutely free. Yes. Perfect. Thank you. Shall I ..." Dial tone, the call was ended.

We had a date and a person. This is awesome news, and for now, I am going to absolutely ignore the fact that our allocated social worker is Doreen, Queen frog from the information evening and somewhere inside me, I was slightly disappointed we did not get a jaunty, overworked team member, ~~more~~ of course we got the haughty shouty one. I need to cancel all my work next Wednesday and make Henri free too, we are on the move!

Wednesday rolled around and we were ready, the house had benefitted from a proper spring clean, and we were confident she wouldn't go in the attic room where we had stashed the contents of the house move that we had not allocated places for yet. In fact, we had moved these boxes from what would be a nursery to the attic room. Made sense to do that, although junk room was indeed a better description than an attic room. Even Digby had had a bath, much to his utter disdain, swim in dirty water, roll in muddy puddles: yes, bathe in clean water: hard no. We waited and at ten thirty, we were arguing over who was going to call the receptionist to ask if there had been a problem when my phone sprang into a loud and tinny version of 'Who Let the Dogs Out'. My latest novelty ringtone. *Might need to change that.*

"I can't access the property. I'm currently located in front of the big church."

"O you mean the Abbey, don't worry Henri is on his way down to get you." I ignored the eye roll from Henri as he shoved his feet into trainers.

I met them at the front door. We exchanged pleasantries, which it seems is all the pleasant Doreen had left in her for the day. She huffed and puffed up our iron spiral staircase and at the top tells us that is too dangerous for children. We don't just need a gate at the top, but soft buffers either side otherwise any child would probably 'break their necks'. I noted it down in the notebook I was carrying alongside a cursory "Yes will add that to my list of to-dos." *Look Doreen at my diligent behaviour, listening intensely and making notes.*

I offered tea but she said we would prefer a coffee. I busied myself making a pot of fresh coffee as Henri made small talk, he is excellent at this being a barber. I started to relax a little, breathing slowed down and shoulders dropped listening to Henri's chitter chatter behind me as the comforting smell of freshly brewing coffee filled the kitchen. I served coffee in our best mugs with an assortment of biscuits. "Would you like milk or cream?"

"Wow, well I can't drink that, it is way too strong. Do you have any normal Nescafe?"

"O goodness, I am sorry I don't, shall I pop to the shop as it really is just on the corner."

"No, think we had better get on, time is short. I'll take a glass of water."

Shoulders resumed position up by my ears, lovely and tense.

"Best start in here then, so this is the kitchen diner?" We nod. "There is a lot to happen in here to make it safe. Kitchen cupboards need child proofing, plug sockets too." She pulls at some drawers and sucks in a breath at the end drawer. "Oooo. No. This is a knife drawer, this is bad. Too accessible. You need to put up a knife holder away from little hands." She scribbles notes and I frantically scribble too. *Bad. Bad. Kitchen. Knives. Sort it. Maybe a refit?* Doreen went on to test the smoke alarms, which thankfully are working, she also pointed out we also have no child-friendly furniture for mealtimes.

She moves herself to the newly fitted bathroom. "Ok, this is all new. Lovely but there is no bath. There needs to be a solution here." *Need a bath, wtf and how do we fit one in this small space?*

We both move to the doorway together and subsequently get wedged, Doreen and I are not small-framed, so the doorway was definitely not going to accommodate us both. She groaned and I swear I smelt pork scratchings on her breath. I backed away. She made her way up the stairs to the attic room.

"We don't need to go up there, it's just a little spare room!" *O God, something may fall on her if she goes in there.*

"Loretta, I do need to see it all."

Right then. "I'll wait in the kitchen, Henri will you go up with Doreen." I am buying time to shake off some irritation. Anyone that uses my name that way makes me immediately spiky. I need to compose myself.

As they descend, I hear, "...completely off limits to a child, so that needs to be sorted out or get a gate at the bottom. Way too dangerous." *Hire a skip to throw stuff away. Buy baby gate. Both.*

On our way to the living room, Doreen comments, "Beautiful balcony. Total no-go for children. That door needs a lock on it."

"It has a lock," I reply. Doreen ignores me, turns to Henri, and says, "Higher." *Replace door.*

"O yes and here three steps up so another child gate." *Buy eleventy billion child gates.*

I lead Doreen to what will be the nursery. She stands in the doorway of the mostly empty room, surveying the space. She doesn't 'hmmm' or utter an 'ooo' or even tut. Silence as she looks about the room. "Well, this will be lovely."

"That's it, nothing I need to do?"

"Well yes obviously as it's not even close to a nursery yet but it's a beautiful-sized room and safely tucked between your bedroom and the living room. This is good." *GOOD!!!! Make it a nursery though. Lots of work.*

We take a seat in the living room, "We do need to address the dog."

"Digby. He is such a good boy, very gentle, everyone loves him."

"Well, in my experience dogs can turn very quickly, you said he was eight years old. You see, adding children in now may upset him as he is pretty long in the tooth. He will need to be analysed by the vet and a report submitted to us so that we can be sure he's not aggressive."

"Are you serious?" Henri's tone is incredulous at this new scathing statement from Doreen, a stretch too far for him. I dared not speak. In fact, if I was Digby, it would have been obvious how I was feeling by emitting a low guttural growl, which Doreen would almost certainly have heard, perhaps with my teeth bared. My fur would be standing on end down my back in utter disgust.

"Deadly. Ok, the application form. It's long and invasive. Are you both ready? We need to contact ex-partners, schools, get you both a full all-over health check including blood work, investigate your finances and make sure you are strong enough not only to endure this process but parenthood. There are nine courses you will need to attend in Bournemouth, or around that area anyway. To be clear, you will both need to attend, and you need to make it a priority. Loretta, you need to get some experience with children, so volunteer somewhere I would, it will look good for you if you do. Right then, I think that's it." Doreen checks her watch as the bongs strike out for midday on the Abbey clock. "O look, nearly lunchtime."

"Ok. I will investigate the volunteering thing, but what about Henri, does he not need experience too?"

"O no, he's a man love. He will probably be at work most of the time."

"Right, is that not a bit sexist?" Henri shoots me a look to not go there. "I mean you know in today's society, females being equal to their male counterparts?"

"Let's just say we all know life doesn't run that way, nor will it ever be so best we just follow the guidelines and get on with it."

Great, so our female-led social working team are sexist against their own gender. Marvellous. This is going to be a fun ride.

"I forgot to say all windows will need locks put on them too. Oh, and whilst I think about it, being situated between two pubs," she sucks air in through her teeth, "Not ideal. Not really. Might be too noisy. I'll look into the noise pollution."
Move house.

Foster To Adopt

A few weeks go by and nothing. Not a word. I don't want to seem like a pushy person by contacting them again but surely, we should have heard something from Doreen by now. Once more I brace myself as I pick up the phone.

"Social Services."

"Adoption department please, Doreen if she is there."

"She's very busy today, I can take a message for her." I close my eyes in mild frustration.

I gently push on, "Can you try her line at all?"

"I could but I won't, what is this regarding?" For the love of all that is holy what is wrong with this woman? I am not trying to get through to the Prime Minister but our allocated social worker.

"We don't want to lose momentum, Doreen came to see us, and we need to start the next step," then I throw in a lie, "She did say I was to get in touch with her, so I am in fact doing what she asked of me." *White lies are ok, yeah?*

The receptionist hesitates for a second, "Doreen told you to ring in and not email? Odd. Ok, alright then, I'll try her line."

The tone rings and rings and just as I think we are about to be rung off; someone picks the phone up all breathy like she's galloped from the other side of the office. "Hello? Sorry I mean Dorset Adoption Department; how can I help you?"

Strike me down she wants to help. "We were wondering if Doreen was available to chat as she came to see us two weeks ago, but we have not heard anything since then."

"Ah. She's eating her lunch, so I won't disturb her." God forbid anyone gets in between Doreen and her sandwich. "Let's see though, what are your names?"

"Loretta and Henri Lupi-Lawrence."

"Found you, Loretta and Henri, got your file." *We have a file, praise be.* "Doreen is not your social worker anymore; she's got too much on. It doesn't say who is replacing her but hang fire, I'll chat to Debbie she may know."

Air punch. Another little dance on the spot. No more Doreen. Why though? Did we do something wrong? Too much on, is she saying we are not important enough to add to her workload? Does she not want more children adopted? Maybe she needs more time to eat. My frustration is tipped over into anger, as overthinking every situation arising is fast becoming my new hobby. The phone clunks onto the desk as she had forgotten to put us on hold, so I am left with background office noises including more than just occasional sighing sounds. I hear her footsteps coming back to the desk, she clears her throat before speaking.

"Ok, so no one is available at the moment to step up." She lowers her voice so I can barely hear her, "It's just all a bit of a mess here currently. Lots of changes. We have some new social workers starting soon. How about I send you the form and get someone to call you when we know? Do you think you could start that on your own for a few weeks? Get ahead of the game."

I huffed and instantly regretted doing so, I didn't want her to think I was a bad person it might affect our chances, so I huffed again and made it sound like a cough. "Absolutely, great. Thanks."

"I will also send over the details of the courses, so you don't fall back on those as they don't happen more than once or twice a year and the new bunch of courses are about to start."

Pru and I met that afternoon and I ranted and let loose all my irritations of our short journey into adoption so far. Pru smiled at me. "You are only just at the beginning; do you think you can overcome these feelings and rationalise what is happening? Acceptance will be key. Don't let this experience become another disappointment. Your challenge for a family is far from over and this part of the process is at the very start. Keep in mind all that you have learnt. Do not spiral." I feel pulled back into the moment. My frustrations at the system versus children in care waiting to be loved, fall away as I try to keep in mind the bigger picture. Deep down, I know that the social services system, however flawed I feel it is, is, in fact, doing good. The staff are all just overworked. The system is just taking the scenic route to finding homes for children that have been let down.

The form was sent in the post. We knew it was the form that had arrived by the huge thud on the doorstep. They were not kidding, this thing was about a hundred and fifty pages long. Alongside the form, was a letter outlining the courses we needed to attend, dates, times, and locations. We needed to email our attendance confirmation.

Things were moving along a little and maybe we were on the boat now instead of waiting on the shore for the boat to arrive. All we needed now was the captain, also known as a social worker to guide us along the river.

Opening up the form, we turned pages upon pages of questions and reports we needed submit. We were instantly completely overwhelmed so put it on the kitchen table to tackle a little later in the week when we had some downtime from work.

Every time I came into the kitchen, it stared at me. Daring me to open its pages and start answering the questions. Questions on who we were, what we did for a career, what money we were earning, who we were going to ask to put down as referees, find ex-partners so they could talk to them, health information, finances, what we did with our days, hobbies, friendships, who had children that we knew, on and on and on. Without guidance, this was not going to be easy to plough through; just getting on with it was not the greatest option. It was massively overwhelming, and it felt like we would be wrestling with a beast.

The first training course we needed to go to was more of a talk. It had been named 'Foster to Adopt', a new form of adoption being trialled. We were back in the same room where we had been introduced to adoption a few months ago. Doreen was once again sitting in the middle of a long table with her open book of notes and an open packet of biscuits in front of her. Sustenance. She was sat between two other people, two adoptive parents. Doreen stood to speak, 'ahemmed' us to silence before uttering, "Good evening, all."

"Foster to Adopt." She let it hang in the air for about twenty seconds and I wondered if she had forgotten where she was and what she was saying. She sprung back into life. "Most potential adopters want a baby. It is a rare thing to have a baby available for adoption. We make decisions to remove children and by then they are usually much older." She stopped talking and surveyed the room, all eyes on her, every single one of us in that room wanting to catch her eye to show her we were listening. Good potential adoptive parents. "Recently we have been looking at the American system where adopters are chosen before a child is born and are even there at the birth. It is still rare in the UK but there are circumstances where this can happen. In fact, it is on the rise where social working teams are able to make orders whilst the mothers are still pregnant. We are calling it Foster to Adopt."

There was some 'oooing' from the room. Satisfied she had whetted our appetites, she continued. "We have trialled this already here in this county, a few times now with huge success." She gestured to the smiling people sitting next to her. "Essentially you need to become foster carers in order to qualify. More training though I am afraid as you will need to be trained to fosterer level."

We all smiled eagerly at her, hoping for her approval to pass us into this new training scheme. "Who here would be interested in becoming a fosterer? Potentially, of course."

The whole room became a sea of hands in the air. It was as if we all had been transported back to school and were certain of the answer to a question the teacher had asked us all.

We learnt that the foster to adopt scheme is where a pregnant mother is deemed unfit from a list of many reasons; drug and alcohol-addicted women, convicted women, mentally unstable women, women that are too young and have no family support, women with abusive history, the list is a long one with the focus firmly placed on the woman. The adoption system heads have researched and reviewed the American adoption system and their processes and seen that in these cases where fostering from birth can give the child a stable home from the beginning of their lives, whilst the courts rule on whether adoption is the best route for the child. Fostering like this also means income for the adoptive parents whilst the adoption orders are granted. All of this sounds ideal to prospective adoptive parents like us. There is a big 'but' coming though. The family courts can very easily overturn the social workers' decisions to have that child removed from the birth mother and the baby will be taken away from the fosterer and handed back the rights to the birth mother. The birth mother and father can fight decisions in court too. It is a risk. The scheme then was a new one and according to Doreen 'on shaky ground.'

"Right then, let's hear from Ben. Ben and his wife were one of the first foster to adopters in Dorset and for them I am pleased to say it has been a resounding success."

Ben was encouraged to stand up as Doreen tapped his shoulder, so he scraped back his chair going a darker shade of pink as he did so. He shifted on his feet looking like he would like to be anywhere else than talking to us.

"Hey all, yup my name is Ben, and we fostered a baby at two days old, he is now one. Our story is simple really, we were in the system as potential adopters, working our way through the courses and we heard there were rumblings of this new scheme Foster to Adopt. We told our social worker that is what we wanted to do and popped ourselves forward for it. Before our baby boy was due to be born, the social working team had already decided the birth mother would not be keeping him as she was merely a child herself, she already had two other children that had been adopted due to her background not being one that was stable or nurturing. Well, let's just put it that way! We were lucky enough to take our baby boy straight home from hospital and begin our parenting journey from there." Ben went on to talk about parenthood and how wonderful it was. Their dreams had come true. He gushed about his son. It moved me and I knew this route is what I also wanted to take. I wanted to take a baby home from a hospital like Ben and his wife. I wanted that.

Mandy then stood up and she too had brought home a baby from hospital, a little girl. Mandy was single, a highflyer in her career but able to take as much time as was needed to bring up her little girl. Another dream family success story.

Warm and fuzzy feelings settled inside me, hope? How do we apply for this? I asked Doreen the question.

"You don't. We choose you based on the outcome of your form and Panel."

"Sorry, what is Panel?" The room sucked in their breath collectively.

"We have spoken about Panel, don't you remember?"

No, you haven't Doreen and we don't have a social worker working with us. I would not forget something that feels quite that important given the reaction in the room, I write stuff down, remember?

Instead, I venture, "Gosh yes sorry, can we have a recap?"

"Ok then," Doreen checks her watch. "Panel is the last part of the adoption process before you move on to actually adopting. You arrive at the Panel room, this one in fact, and there will be a Panel of around twelve people. Social working heads of department, a few professionals like a doctor and psychiatrists, county councillors, and previous adopters. People that are qualified to assess your application form and ask you all the right questions. You will be interviewed separately and then together. If you pass this, you are passed to go ahead and adopt a child."

A loaded silence fell in the room. ThePanel sounded to me like it might be worse than an A-level oral in German at school whilst hopping on one leg, it felt like working towards this final step involved a leap of faith. A chill made its way down my spine as I realised those people on the Panel were going to be deciding on our future. What do councillors know about adoption or how worthy we are or are not to adopt. The mere mention of the word Panel and clearly it throws all of us potential adopters into the lion's den and it weighs heavy on all our minds.

Doreen breaks the silence by opening a Kit Kat and snapping the chocolate fingers off before shoving them in her mouth. "That's it for tonight folks," firing biscuit wafer and chocolate over those closest to her.

Training Begins

Unlike being pregnant, watching a beautiful round baby bump grow, downloading an app that gives you week-by-week updates on how big the baby is growing and likening it to different food types, or maybe bonding with other NCT mamas and papas, training for adoption is quite different. Instead of pitching up to a room of protruding bellies, coffee, or tea on offer, maybe some biscuits, lighthearted chatter about how the baby is now the size of an avocado and which pram will they be getting, potential adopters get to sit in a darkened, cold room on even colder uncomfortable red and green plastic chairs or if you are lucky a soft low chair that is heavily stained with God only knows what. Best not to think about it. We will not be chatting about bumps and pushchairs but more the business of why children are taken from their homes, why we have to jump through more hoops than dogs at Crufts, what abuse looks like in children, how this abuse is manifested, how to deal with an abused child, mental, physical and sexual abuse, child hunger, behaviour patterns. You know the juicy stuff.

Back in my sessions with Pru, I voiced my sadness at this, how I don't get to bond with other expectant mamas that start parenting not as they birth a child but at the maternity wear section in M&S and laughing at not being able to do shoelaces up at full term. We made no NCT friends. We sat in a lifeless room with mostly stony-faced over worked social workers drilling us on the most likely trauma triggers that will be inherent in a child if they come from a violent background. I have not really wanted to admit that every time I see a new parent pushing a pram or with a baby on their lap, I turn my head away as fast as I can because it hurts. Why can't this be me? Why didn't I have a little baby to push around or hold gleefully in my arms, smudging its nose and cooing at it? I would swallow my grief down and rush home or to the toilet and spill the tears silently taking huge gulps of air in to calm me down. I worked hard to resolve this new level of grief by culminating in a conclusion. Finally, a real endpoint, I begin to realise that that kind of thinking is very unhelpful to where we are on this journey. I needed to learn to embrace our own kind of parental training. Hard as it is, that is the fact of it. I am not pregnant; I am adopting a child that needs a loving home not one fraught with violence and neglect. We work through this week after week until one session I realise I am ok with it. More than ok, I feel like the shackles of grief are loosening as I finally accept that I do not need to be pregnant to be a mother. *Acceptance is how I unlock the padlock and I have the key now.*

I left Pru that day feeling light-footed, I had been truly released. I walked back towards the apartment, stopping to sit on the lawn outside the Abbey to soak in some sunshine, where Henri joined me. I beamed at him as he strode over to me, his eyes resting on mine.

"I am ok. I am really ok with it. I think I've found peace. You know that sad, jealous part of my grief babe, I've worked it through. I've seen three mamas with babies on the way back from Pru's and instead of turning away from them I smiled at the little ones, and it gave me joy not pain. One baby gurgled at me, it was cute, I feel, I don't know, a bit different, lighter somehow."

I didn't realise it but in that moment between us, tears had sprung and were coursing down my face, the happiest tears, those of pure relief. I looked into Henri's eyes and his were watery too, we hugged for a long time. Henri whispered into my ear, "I knew you could do it. I am so proud of you."

We lay on the lush green lawn gazing up at the blue sky and passing clouds, holding hands chatting about the work I had done, how I had arrived here to this point, all the while identifying clouds that looked like animals. I asked him how he was for the first time knowing I had space to hold him and support him. I apologised again for neglecting his own grief, he was feeling all this too, my eyes were open. A new sensation coursed through my body and with it every cell in my body was alert, I had woken up from the zombie-like existence I had been living and was really ready to start to embrace my life just as it was. I felt a real rush of love for Henri, without him it doesn't bear thinking about.

On our way to our first training session in a town we had to drive an hour to get to, we felt nervous. We arrived in the car park of the old red brick council building that if I did not know better looked like it was a multi-story car park. The ivy was taking over the outer walls of the building, it crept up and around drainpipes and windowsills. Weeds growing at ground level giving the building a kind of green skirting board. The windows were a dirty grey and covered in bird poo. The signs on the building, green with age and neglect. "Once more unto the breech babe." We climbed out of the car and buzzed to gain access to the building. We stood under grey skies, huddled together against the cold moisture in the air. I shivered as raindrops started to beat down on us.

"Ooo come in, come in. Sorry I made you wait, just me today so bear with me whilst I turn on the heating, bit nippy in here, eh? Just got to prep the handouts and tables. Others are here, do join them. The kitchen is over there for a cuppa. Might have to wash cups, pretty sure there is milk in date lurking in the fridge. O and the loo is right outside the room. I am Janet by the way." Janet was a thin woman with glasses balanced on the end of her pointed nose. She wore a thin olive-green jumper over a shirt and paired that with formal navy blue straight-legged trouser. Trainers on her feet, which I suspected were to get her to where she needed to go a little faster. Her hair short and white, with small diamond earrings glittering in her ears, a little hint that she is more than her sensible clothing would suggest.

We walked into the oblong room at the end of the corridor which closely resembled a classroom but with no children's artwork hanging on the walls. The same uniform plastic chairs from the other council building placed in a semi-circle. Only two remained empty at the end of the row which we claimed. A few of the other couples were nursing chipped mugs of hot liquid and some sipping from cardboard takeaway cups. We had not been that organised, well in truth I had made us a couple of coffees, but I had left them on the side in the kitchen in my haste to leave on time. No one was chatting so we sat and whispered out hellos and smiles. I busied myself getting out a notebook and pens, Henri crossed his arms, sighed and threw his legs under the chair. He hated stuff like this, he was missing a day at work and anything resembling a school set up propelled him backwards into the early 1980s. We waited as Janet shuffled papers and muttered notes to herself before finally looking up with a sigh, "We had best begin. We have only five hours and lots to cram in."

Wait, what? Five hours! I looked at Henri and mouthed 'Digby' and grimaced. We had left Digby at home all comfy gently snoozing on his bed, but we thought it would only take the journey plus one hour tops. My mind busied itself with trying to figure out who could go in and check on him, take him for a loo break when Henri's elbow dug into my ribs. I realised everyone was facing me waiting for a reply to a question I had not heard.

"O yes, hello! I'm Loretta, Henri's wife."

"Yes, Henri has told us that bit, we wanted to know what you think will make you a good adoptive mother, your thoughts on that at this stage in the process."

Caught off guard, I smiled, babbling, "Well you know, I am, I mean, I have a dog. It's the same isn't it really? Dogs and kids?!" I knew it was wrong as soon as the sentence had slipped from my lips.

"Not really no, Loretta. You can't just walk a child, give him or her some food and let the child sleep all day. Nor can you go out and leave the child on their own!" Janet took out her pad and wrote down some notes. Her smile had disappeared. "Ok let's ask John the same question, what will make you a great adoptive dad?"

Bugger. Strike one already. I felt shame, *I was joking, it was a joke Janet!* Ok I was distracted and lost track of the conversation. My bad. I internalised the shame and I could feel little pinpricks at the back of my eyes where tears threatened to fall. I have this thing with being misunderstood, it happens a lot. Too much. I sometimes don't manage to make the best decisions or find the right words on the spur of the moment. Then I feel judged by it. I guess I am just not that clever at thinking on my feet. I joke when I feel awkward, it's a design flaw. I look at my lap until the feeling passes. Henri's hand had reached across to rest on my arm. He squeezed it and as I snuck a look up, he smiled until I looked away again mentally tucking away another lesson. *Do not make jokes, put that side of you away in these sessions.*

It was going to be a long five hours.

We learned about the typical cycle a child can go through when they are taken from their birth homes. What trauma can come with these children and how parenting for adoption is very different to parenting children who are living with their birth families. We mostly came to understand what attachment is, how this affects all children, how this is the single most important part of the adoption process but also how this can take up to a year or three to fall into place, sometimes longer.

Attachment, in short, is where inside birth families this happens almost immediately, the baby is birthed and then placed on the mother or father, the baby senses this is their safe place, as was the womb which kickstarted this bond nine months ago. Then attachment continues through that bond with parenting, a child will attach to a parent's behaviour and mannerisms, mimicking their parents as they learn their way in life through them. For example, when a mother comes to the aid of a child as he or she has fallen overgrazing a knee, the child learns empathy, kindness, and trust. In most cases this is all positive but in cases where a child learns anger, or resentment, or solitude, then the child can mimic the learned negative attached behaviours carrying this forward into their life.

With adoption, you must create this bond without the aid of a womb or birthing process, and it almost certainly will not be immediate, it is something that must be nurtured, and existing learned attached behaviours need to be unpicked with new positive behaviours replacing the old. It can take years and attachment success really depends on the individual child's history before removal from the birth home.

Armed with a list of books to buy on this subject, we said our goodbyes and shuffled out to the car in silence, all of us exhausted from the mental fireworks now popping off in our brains. So much information to digest. I felt a little numbness against the creeping realisation that some of these couples will walk away now choosing a different life. As we reached the doors leading to the car park, I could hear mummering from other couples, "Bloody hell didn't know adoption was going to be this hard," and "Up to two years to attach. That can't be right."

We decompressed as we drove home, Henri reached for my thigh resting his hand there as I drove. "You, ok?"

"Yup. It was a lot though, wasn't it? I mean I wasn't expecting it to be a walk in the park but there is so much to consider, we really do have so much to learn. Attachment feels like this huge thing we will need to conquer, and we won't know if we can do it until we have a child, I guess. We have it in us though, don't we? I think we do. What's another hurdle to jump over after all we've jumped so far?"

"Of course we can, you and I will learn this together and just go out and do it. Don't we always?" His reassurance doing wonders soothing my overworked brain. "Stop trying to cover up your quirks, I love them." He smiled at me, then started to laugh.

The training kept coming thick and fast as we dived deep into the world of adoption. Some training days were easier than others. One Sunday, we had to just take a sheet of paper and draw us in the centre of the page and write the names of the people closest to us around our own names, then those next closest and then associates we could lean on in the outer circle. The purpose of this was to show us what kind of support network we realistically had. Another day we learned solely about disabilities in children and how to parent with them. Autism, ADHD, ADD, Down Syndrome, ME, impairments, epilepsy, hyperactivity, dyslexia, dyspraxia, high functioning autism, Asperger syndrome, dyscalculia, pervasive development disorder, sensory processing disorder. When I asked why we were learning this because realistically, any child anywhere could live with one or another disability from the list, we were told that many children in care had been neglected because of these disabilities which led the birth parent to not cope, and as adopters picking up the pieces we needed to be prepared.

Some days we would just listen to endless adoption stories, some successful and others that were not. Some adopters had a fight on their hands with schools, others had to admit defeat and hand the children back to social services. All of it quite daunting as we turn the questions onto ourselves, would we be successful, what about if we are not and have to make a heartbreaking decision? As the training bus rumbled on, I noticed we lost a good handful of potential adopters, and the training rooms were emptier at each next session.

I read the recommended books when Henri was at work. So many books to plough through. These books were laborious and heavy, I quite often had to re-read pages as my mind had walked off in a huff over how intense the material was, or I had simply fallen asleep.

The penny was dropping, and I was starting to get it, adoption needed much more than giving a loving and nurturing home to a child, it was more than that. It was walking their path too alongside parenting. It was being on high alert for the small signs of trauma creeping in, or understanding that a tantrum could mean so much more than 'the terrible twos' and the best way to deal with one was to get on their level and let them go at it, give them the time to scream in the supermarket aisle, sitting with them on the floor until they could allow themselves to fold into your open arms.

Henri worked, I read, we went to training, I had therapy, we set plans in motion for the new business. Another new normal had developed for us.

We had heard not a peep from the adoption department, just as we were giving up hope of any guidance from anyone in social services, Louisa walked into our lives. She was the torch we needed in our cave, with her arrival came a calm and reassuring perspective. She smiled a lot; her smiles were not forced they were genuine as her eyes matched the curve in her mouth. She listened to everything we had to say, and we had a lot to say as we had had no one for guidance and support for such a long time. She was taller than me with shoulder-length soft grey curly hair that sat on her shoulders, she wore lots of colour, floral prints on long skirts or dungarees topped off with a soft doughy woolen knit. Her face softly creased as she smiled in all the right places like she had had a lot of laughter in her life. She was a mother to two girls in secondary school and a wife to someone she loved deeply. Louisa's voice was softly spoken too, when she spoke it felt like the warmth from the first fire of the season spreading heat into every corner, comforting, encouraging. Her deep blue eyes always searched for mine as she spoke, when I spoke, she looked at me so directly like she felt every word I was saying, understood my pain and longing. She heard me. She was not just our social worker but a kindred soul, a companion, a confidante.

She had confessed during our afternoon together that she really disliked how the adoption system worked, she thought parts of it were archaic, but she drummed it home that no matter what anyone thought of the process, it was what we needed to do to get through to Panel. Louisa had transferred over to this department from being a social worker assigned to the children taken into care. She knew what the children needed in adopters, and these children, she told us needed people just like Henri and I. She spoke gently about their pain and explained that unlike the 1960s when children were given up at birth due to being illegitimate or unwanted, these children now are being taken away from parents that are doing them harm. From adults that should know better. Child abuse is happening all around us. The abuse can be varied from parents just not engaging with their children, allowing them watch TV all day, or starving the children, or beating them or worse. Mostly, abuse was learnt from their own childhood attachments. It was a cycle of neglect. Poverty also has a huge hand in child abuse. She added that the foster homes were at bursting point. We were sobered from that initial conversation, but we finally felt supported, we were more determined than ever to move forward and give a child a good, wholesome home. A loving one. One where love replaces abuse.

Of the many things during our initial chat that we talked about Louisa explained to us that most first-time adopters wanted only to adopt a baby and at a stretch they will consider a toddler under three years old. Under three, because it is believed that most trauma that is experienced early on enough can be reversed with love, care, kindness and understanding as they are so young and impressionable. This was true for us too, to have a family where everyone else starts, at the beginning. Children over seven years old tend to get passed from foster home to foster home as they are deemed too damaged to be adopted which very oddly reminded me of the children's game of 'pass the parcel,' the parcel never really landing anywhere it can settle before it is ripped apart and sent on its merry way again.

"We want a baby too or a toddler but yeah, a baby. This makes me feel guilty and sad for the older children in care but if I am honest, I don't think I could cope with an older child as I have no experience with children really. Well at all. My nephews grew up when we lived away from here, so I never had the opportunity to be a hands-on aunt. Gosh, even that makes me feel terrible. Does that make us bad adoptees already?"

Louisa's smile spread across her face, reaching her eyes, reassuring us, "Of course not, I can already see you have so much love to give, and this is not something we should be worrying about now. So many adopters start this way and change their minds; some don't. All children just need good homes. I will get you to where you need to be for Panel and once you are approved, we will chat about this again. Let's get this form underway and see if we can make up some lost time. You need to make a doctor's appointment for the medicals. They know what to do, nothing to worry about height, weight, healthy heart, and bloods need to be taken. I will take you step by step through this form. Fill in the first section as best you can, it's about your history and relationships. Bit by bit we will eat up this form to get you to that Panel fully ready. Bite-size chunks will make it more manageable." She smiled again.

There is nothing like having someone other than your husband to hold your hand as you walk across the hot coals on a specific path of life. With IVF we had no one to talk to about our baby loss, our continual failures. No one who had failed too and had given up all hope. The adoption journey has so far not been as smooth as I would have liked, who could we ask for help from? All the social workers we had met before Louisa were shut down, too busy, angry and frustrated, underpaid, and it would seem quite hungry.

She hugged me as she left and held my shoulders, "Believe in yourself. I already believe in you. You will make great parents." She waved goodbye as she crossed the road and up the steps out of view.

"Well, I do believe that we finally have someone on our side." Someone that had shown us some kindness, someone that had listened to every word we had to say. We finally had our first break in this journey to a family. It felt like the first jigsaw puzzle piece had slotted into place.

Save The Worst Until Last

The very last training session had come around at last. It was a hot Sunday in June, and we were back inside the old red brick council building that smelt of damp and despair. It had become familiar now though and we stopped at a friendly Eastenders-style café we had found along the canal path and grabbed two large takeaway coffees and some sweet pastry treats. Once again, we were back for another five-hour stint but this time with a speaker from the NSPCC.

After so much training, we had become dab hands at the entry systems and chatted much more freely with the other remaining potential adopters. We were one couple out of six that had made it this far, originally, we were a group of twenty-four couples. The room was still cold but a more welcome relief this time from the already rising temperature outside. The atmosphere was a jolly one, we had come so far since the first session in February, a whole two seasons had passed us by, and this was finally the last training session. Everyone was feeling that there was light at the end of the training tunnel.

Buoyed by the fact that we now had Louisa working alongside us, we had made it this far, and we had made a start on the form. We were on catch-up, but Louisa was confident we could get it in by the end of the summer.

Janet was waiting for our guest speaker outside in the car park. I noted that she seemed a little jumpy today, on edge.

I was chatting to a couple that had already submitted their form, I was frisking them for hints and tips when a familiar voice entered the room before she did. "Ok everyone let's take a seat, shall we? I am just going to run through what is happening today before I hand over." Doreen.

I eye rolled, inwardly of course, I was getting good at not allowing the real me out during training hours. I beamed at her; *look Doreen we are still here!* but she didn't look in my direction. We all found seats. "So today, we saved the best until last. Or the worst depending on how you look at it. This is the session most people find the toughest. It is hard-hitting but we need you to understand the reality of adoption, what came before for many children in our care system. Why children are placed in care. If you need to leave the session at any time, please take a small break in the kitchen, we understand you may need to take breaks today."

There was a seismic shift in the room, the atmosphere had dropped like stone, and everyone was very much sobered. Doreen had given us a stern warning and we all heeded it. Breaking the silence was Janet tripping along the corridor, "Just through here, yes really hot today, yes, room at the end as usual."

In front of Janet was a short lady with even shorter hair. She wore blue jeans turned up at the ankle, she had paired them with a loose white shirt neatly tucked into the belted waistband with polished black Doc Martin boots. Thick round black framed glasses sat on her bare face, and she was carrying a tatty, brown, leather briefcase. Her voice was low, serious. Her smile was a thin line. She observed us in the same way we were observing her whilst Janet busied herself sorting out the desk and asking her where she wanted the chair placed before Doreen and Janet exited the room.

"Hi, everyone. My name is Sam and I work at the NSPCC. I am going to dive straight in. My work is not pretty or gentle to be honest. For example, I was one of the leading team members working on the Jimmy Saville case, which I hasten to add is far from over and we are still processing. There are more than two hundred victims being processed on top of the already known four hundred and fifty or so. Anyway, that gives you a hint at what is coming today so I want to reiterate, just like Doreen and Janet said, if you want to take a breather, please do, I am here to educate you on what children could have gone through, some of it is extreme and other parts of it less so but all of it should never have happened to a child."

Silence fell over us, gone was the excitement that this was our last training session. No one moved or spoke. I snuck a look at Henri whose face was set into an expression of concern, I caught his eye, he didn't smile to reassure me, he just took my hand and turned back to face Sam.

Sam had pulled forward a whiteboard. "Ok, let's begin with childhood. Shout out some fun and happy memories from your childhood."

"Puddle jumping," said Cathy with relief in her voice now that we were talking about happier things.

"Christmas and birthdays!" Chris shouted.

"Baking with my mama, reading on my grandpa's knee whilst we ate Murray mints," I ventured.

Lots more suggestions come out, flying kites, caravan holidays in the rain, being tucked into bed at night with a kiss, steaming bowls of sweet homemade porridge on a Saturday morning, Sunday morning muddy rugby training sessions. Sam was nodding and enthused by our responses. We were all almost giddy with the memories that had filled up our own childhoods.

"That's great," Sam pointed to the full sheet on the board. She smiled her flatline smile looking at each of us one at a time. Turning to the board, she grabbed the sheet of paper, tore it off and screwed the paper into a ball before throwing it as far as she could against the wall behind us. With a dull thud it hit the dirty window, bounced off the filing cabinets as it fell, then landed on the barely there blue carpet.

Collectively we sucked in our breath. "Forget all of that. That is not the childhood that any child in the care system would recognise. That happiness, security, trust, and love you all felt they will never have felt it."

I shifted in my seat, pulled my hand from Henri's as he was holding it so tight it was starting to go numb. I broke the uncomfortable silence that reigned in the room. "That is so shocking," I spoke but to no one in particular, I had an overwhelming need to sever the tense atmosphere that had built up. Everyone else murmured in agreement. Sam's act of ripping off the paper, screwing it up and throwing it across the room was as powerful as her words that followed the act itself.

"Yeah, I get that but that is the best way for me to introduce you to this session. It will be shocking. It will be upsetting. Only one per cent of children in care have been voluntarily given up, maybe less than that. The majority of kids in the care system have come from abusive homes where adults have failed them, adults that should never have been left alone to bring up children. These kids have seen things that no child should ever bear witness to, they have been put through hell. I am going to set out some examples now, please ask questions if you need to."

What came next is nothing that I expected when I was getting ready for this session this morning. It is the stuff of nightmares and all of it happening all over our country, in every country around the world. Sam spoke at length about the Jimmy Saville case holding nothing back. His victims went through life not being believed, heard, or protected from a monster.

I too now believe in monsters.

"I have been working closely with a family that has had three children, all those children have been taken away and placed in care. The mum got herself pregnant again recently. Each time she is pregnant we go through the same process of assessment. I know this couple well now and they know me; I walk into the room and the dad will swear at the sight of me. I asked him this the last time I saw him, 'What makes this pregnancy different this time around?' They both pleaded their cases that they had been better lately, no drugs, some alcohol, and definitely no real arguments. So, I said, 'No arguments Billy? Are you sure about that?' Billy told me they had had a few but nothing like how it used to be. 'Do you still get angry Billy? Like before?' Absolutely not he reassured me, but he added, 'Sometimes she just winds me up you know?' 'Ok, how about you show me Billy?'"

Sam moved forward to the chair sitting out of place in the middle of the room. She moved it to one side.

"So, I asked him, 'Show me Billy. Your level of anger, just show me. If you hit the chair here as if it was Sharon or one of your children, would it move much?' He showed me." Without warning Sam kicked the chair so far across the room it took flight from the floor and landed with an almighty crash on top of another set of stacked plastic chairs. We all flinched. My heart was in my throat. "That was when we made the order for the child to be taken away at birth. Billy claimed that that level of strength was only a tap. That brute force you just witnessed me do to the chair, was just a 'tap' to Billy. Imagine real hot impulsive anger. Billy does not understand his strength but more than that he does not care, he does not see anything wrong with violence. Sharon is under a spell with him despite her scars and permanent sets of bruises all inflicted by his 'taps'. Whilst the order was a simple one the harder job for us was keeping her safe, so no harm came to her unborn child."

Cathy spoke, her voice a whisper, "Why does she not leave? Can you not take her away from him? Get an injunction?"

"We do not have the power to do that, she is an adult of sound mind. There is nothing we can do for her."

Cathy left the room crying followed by Amanda some minutes later. I sat there numb with disbelief. I was starting to feel a bit sick. My breath caught in my chest. My throat was painful as I gulped back the impulse to cry for Sharon and her unborn child, her three other children. Cathy and Amanda came back in with red eyes and tissues.

"People are inherently cruel guys. I have seen with my own eyes the bruising, the terror in a child's eyes. I work closely with social services and the children in care to help them, get them to safety. Last week I took a mother and her six-month-old baby girl away from her family home and husband in one of the most horrific cases I ever had to deal with. The mother called our helpline with no idea what to do or where to turn. Her husband appeared to anyone looking in, a loving family man, in a steady job working as an accountant, living in a lovely townhouse. They had a mortgage and a good family and friends' network around them. Normal life. Or so it seemed until she discovered something that was so abhorrent, she was left with no choice but to act on it. She found out all by chance."

I scraped my chair back and as quickly as I could, escaped the room. Pushing open the toilet door I made it just before I vomited. I wretched into the toilet until I had nothing left. I closed the door and sat on the toilet lid. *Surely this wasn't real life. What kind of people were living among us? How has this happened to humanity, how are we capable of it?* I silently wept for the unborn baby, the three children, Sharon, the mother of the six-month-old but mostly, the baby girl. I was in no hurry to go back in. I felt agonised for all the children going through torturous childhoods. I took my time, blew my nose, wiped my eyes, washed my face in the freezing water from the tap before I reluctantly made my way back into the room. Henri stood and walked over to me putting his arm around me escorting me back to our seats.

Sam told us yet more stories, one about a little boy in a happy home, he was seven years old and in a seaside town for a day trip with his mother. He needed the toilet whilst they were walking through the beautiful, lush flowering gardens which lead to the sandy beach. His mother found a public toilet and beckoned him into the ladies' side but being seven years old now he wanted to use the male toilet. She waited outside the door. After three or so minutes she moved forward to call her son's name moving out of the way of a man exiting. The boy had been inappropriately touched within just those three minutes, in that toilet. Silenced by the hand of his attacker covering his mouth. Sam repeated that nowhere is safe from predators. Nowhere.

I tried to switch my brain off and think of household chores I needed to do when we got home, I had heard enough. The session was too long and more than uncomfortable but as we headed towards the end of it, I fully understood why it was so necessary. Learning how to parent and help children carrying this level of trauma, how to wade through their sludge to get to the heart of them is something we all needed to learn as adopters. Something we must face given the statistics of children in care.

For the first time on this journey, I felt privileged to be in this position, I wasn't envious of cosy NCT meetings anymore. We were not being taught how to swaddle a baby, or breastfeed over posh coffee and bumps but more how to be a life raft in rough sea, a safe reliable port in the storm that children in care had imposed on them. It is an odd feeling to finally feel at peace with shattered dreams. In fact, shattered dreams become something else, they transform into a life we were not supposed to be living, no longer the dream. That is why it has always been so hard. I see it now. Fighting against the force of what was not meant for us. We were never meant to have our own children genetically; it was never meant to be that way. This path in this cold room with thin blue carpet, stained chairs, and an odd smell of sour milk was exactly where we were supposed to be.

Sam wrapped up her session as Doreen came in swinging a Waitrose bag of food for her lunch followed by Janet on her heel. "Lunch now, I think. How was it all folks? It's a tough one that session. Take half an hour and decompress. Thanks Sam, can Janet make you a coffee?"

No one really spoke as we filed out into the sunshine. I had forgotten it was warm and sunny outside, it truly felt like it was winter inside that building where we learnt about the grim, dark world of abuse in children. I was grateful for the sun on my skin. I stood still and tipped my head to the sky, warming up my bones and letting the light flood back in. "Let's get food," Henri took my hand. "Shall we talk about that?"

"Yes, no. Maybe not now. How do you feel?"

"I feel like I have been a very naïve man throughout my life. In my wildest nightmares I did not realise this kind of thing was real. I mean the..." He tailed off and shook his head.

"Let's get some wine from Vineyards later and we can pull that apart over a glass away from here." We reached the entrance to Waitrose, and we split into different aisles to seek out our lunches. Henri found me in the chiller aisle shelves, staring at the array of different salads on offer. "Hey, you ok?"

"No." Fresh tears covered my face as I silently sobbed amongst office workers, leaning in to get their lunches. "It's so horrendous. I can't just choose a salad and get on with my life. I don't want to go back to the training room."

"I get it, but we have too. We are nearly done for the day and then training is complete. We've got this and we can feel the impact of it later, at home with Digby snuggled in with us and that glass of wine."

"I am not hungry."

"Me either." Henri put his sandwich in amongst the salads, grabbed my hand and took me back out into the sunshine.

The afternoon session to endure was just one hour long and we had been promised a lighter topic. Janet handed each of us a sheet of paper. On it was a list of disabilities and tick boxes. The task was simple. Names at the top and tick which disabilities we would be willing to accept in an adopted child. Turns out I could be shocked again that day.

Rumbles of noise and conversations started as we scraped chairs, moved bags, and turned to confide in our partners. "What the fuck?" I mouthed to Henri.

"This is too much." I could see the stress in his face. We just looked at each other and then the sheet. The couple next to us were discussing whether having a child that was blind would be better than a deaf child having already agreed they would have a child with Down Syndrome and/or ADHD. I felt appalled by it.

I stood. "Does it matter Doreen?" She looked up at me quizzically and the room looked up from their hushed discussions. "I mean I feel this is crazy, will it go against us as prospective adopters if we don't tick any box or just the disabilities we think we can deal with? It's nuts. Surely, we will just get to the point of adopting and love the child no matter what, regardless of disability?"

"Well, Loretta, it does matter to us, to the children. Usually they all have something; what do you think you can cope with?"

"No child is going to be perfect but to be picking from a list feels well, archaic." *You had to open your mouth and ruin it didn't you*? O well, in for a penny, in for a pound. "And wrong. It feels wrong." There. I said it. Here I go with my opinions again. Henri shoots me a look of pride.

"Does it? If you cannot cope with any of those on the list, it is ok to not tick a box."

"Is it ok? How will it look on Panel day? Heartless? Will I have limited my ability to mother and love by not ticking any boxes but in truth I don't know how I would cope until I am presented with it?"

The room had now fallen completely silent. Cathy spoke up in support, "I agree honestly, I am not comfortable with this form either." I thanked her for speaking up by giving her a warm smile, I had come to like Cathy. She was the wife of a vicar with four children of their own, they were in the adopting process because they had room to welcome another child into their family. She wasn't preachy, but more earthy and in tune with the stars. I liked that, the social workers didn't she told me, referring to her as 'a bit too woo woo and wacky.'

Doreen sighed heavily and shook her head. "How about we end the session here, you guys take the form home and have a longer think about it? Submit it with your application form. Hmm?" Doreen slurped down the rest of her tea, stood up and smoothed out wrinkles from sitting too long in a linen dress. "Any more questions?" She did a cursory glance over the group resting her eyes on me whilst raising an eyebrow.

I shook my head, forced out a smile, and shoved the paper in my bag. I was so ready to leave that old red brick building behind me. We said our goodbyes, wished everyone good luck and almost ran from the building to the car.

The Application Form

It had been around a month since we left the council training building behind us. Life had moved at such a fast pace that we could barely keep up. As well as diligently filling in parts of the form, question by question, we also got the keys to our new shop on the high street. We got stuck into painting the walls and sanding old floors back to their former pre-glued glory, found a manager for our old shop and applied for loans and grants to kick-start the new business. Pru and I had decided to go to bimonthly meetings as I was starting to feel stronger from within myself. Puzzle pieces started falling into place, sometimes with forgiveness and other parts with just acceptance that that was just how it was.

The nursery was painted a pale light yellow, a reflection of the room where I did my healing work in Pru's house. To me, this was the colour of calm, safety, being held. I had started to buy things for the room, a lampshade, pictures for the walls, wall stickers with the fun circus theme I imagined last year, a cute rabbit-shaped rug, a vintage cabinet that could double as a changing unit that I cleaned up and painted, books, and a bookshelf. Louisa told me to 'hold my horses' when I announced to her that I had bought a Winnie the Pooh step and toilet training seat. I knew she was right it was too early, but my spirit was a little crushed regardless.

The medical reports had come back with no blemishes on them other than highlighting my anxiety. My old nemesis anxiety loved getting a mention, as when I read the report, I could feel a congratulatory tightening of my chest. It was noted that I was in therapy but not on medication. We had sent out an email to contact Henri's ex-wife. Did I mention he was once married for all of about five minutes? A short and definitely not sweet marriage where I think both were relieved when it was over, anyway social services wished to talk to her, this was making Henri jumpy as they had not ended on the best of terms plus, we had to locate her and rumour had it she was living overseas. The friends and family forms were filled in ready for the social workers to call them and make appointments to talk about us. Our vet practice had submitted their report praising Digby and his calm, non-confrontational temperament. Proud dog mama moment for me, as if he had passed a bunch of GCSEs. The house had been signed off as child-friendly after putting in the work to make sure it was a safe environment. The car had been looked over and approved. Our choices of nurseries and schools noted. We answered what religion the child would have, signed a committal to Letterbox, this is what adopters are asked to sign up for when adopting, basically you are accepting that you need to write to the birth family every year to update them on your adopted child's progress. It is a hard pill to swallow as it is always that once-a-year threshold that reminds you that you are not left alone to be a normal family living out our days. The birth family can also send you letters around this time too. We pledged that the child would have English as their primary language. The form stating which disabilities filled in despite how much it left a bitter taste in our mouths. Crossing the t's and dotting those i's.

The majority of this paperwork application for a family was nearly at an end.

We had arrived at the tricky financial section of the form, did we have enough money to give a child a home, what were our income streams, could we afford for one of us to take off a year, how could we afford that, what were our outgoings, any savings or property, what was our exact amount of debt, to whom and what was the APR %, did we have any credit cards, was the car paid for, what were the details of our mortgage, on and on. No stone was going to be left unturned, they were drilling down including asking us to submit a year's worth of bank statements with justification notes on all our outgoings and income.

We had become stuck, drowning in numbers so we called in our backup in Louisa for a coaching chat.

Louisa had become a beacon of light to us, our personal lighthouse on the rough unknown seas. She mentored us through what we needed to do, what the social working heads wanted to see, which boxes needed to be ticked. Louisa explained it was mandatory that one person needed to be at home with the adopted child for a year to make sure attachment was given the best chance, just as a new mother or father would do having a child of their own. The biggest difference being that maternity and paternity leave is recognised but adoption leave is largely not, at the time of our application anyway. Just another bump in the road to adopting. We needed to prove we were financially sound when one person took a year off to parent. It was a crucial part of the application.

Henri and I set about working out how this was going to be possible, we may have over-egged the income by a wide margin. Louisa pointed out that we would be working from a new business model and how were we to know, plus we planned on selling our other business for a lump sum income. I say *we*, but Henri did most of this part of the application.

Finance is not a strong point of mine (understatement), there is this constant push and pull with Henri and I, I like to spend with abandon, paying not a jot of notice to the sums in (or not in) the bank account and Henri is the saver and frugal part of our marriage. It mostly works.

When I was at school I was flummoxed by numbers. Numbers swam across the page and switched places often stacking on top of one another, I had no idea how to capture them and come forth with the correct answer. More often than not I would read numbers back to front. I struggled and was inevitably in the bottom classes for math lessons. I failed my GCSE math with an undignified 'ungraded', so my parents bought me extra tuition for the retake, and I still only managed to scrape a D grade. Still, I was very happy with that grade, even if no one else was. In my twenties, money seemed to just dissolve. I never had lessons on how to budget or save money. I was hopeless. Only now do I recognise that I have dyscalculia. Asking me about finances throws me into a mild panic, spins my head around and my stress levels hit the roof. Give me words any day.

I watched Henri sit and work out the profits and income and then the outgoings, observed his predictions for the financial future, marvelled at his planning for new income to give us a boost, and gawped at the savings I didn't know were there. Slowly he gave me the answers to put into the form. Henri doesn't do forms so this is where I can excel! Balance.

The form was finally done. Finished. Ready. Tick. We were ready. Tick. We whizzed it over to Louisa for the once-over. She booked a date to go over the form and talk to us about the interviews that had been scheduled with some family members, the ex-wife who had been located and some friends.

Nerves would have kicked in a little, but we were so busy getting the new barbershop ready for opening. The floors were now stained with deep mahogany oil, the barber chairs had arrived and been assembled, the silver on them gleaming in the light. The enormous mirrors double my height had also arrived and been delicately placed in. My little office was set up in the staff room. The vintage rug we had bid for had arrived from eBay; two rows of vintage cinema chairs found in a flea market skillfully installed by a carpenter. Freshly painted walls and skirtings. Our beautifully painted sign mounted above the entrance doorway. Nearly ready for opening.

The interviews of our referees were being done by Doreen, I had pre-warned our friends and family they needed instant coffee and some custard creams, a cake, if possible, to make the right first impression. They all said they were 'grilled' but otherwise the interviews went ok. The phone call to Henri's ex-wife also went well, it turns out she is so happy in her new life in Denmark with her small children that she seems to have forgotten how acrimonious their spilt was. She gave Henri a glowing report. Henri was stunned. I was relieved.

The date made to go through the form with Louisa happened to be the same date we opened the shop for the first time. Louisa was unfazed and came to the shop half an hour before it opened its doors. Louisa and I sat in the cinema chairs in the bright shop window with Digby resting after his long romp through the fields at our feet as Henri paced in front of us joking, he felt like he was in that sketch with Adrian Edmondson and Rik Mayall in Bottom when they started a business which was doomed to fail. I went over the form with Louisa whilst Henri swept up hair he had not yet cut.

"Ok Louisa, give it to me, what do I need to change?" There had to be a load of edits.

"It's good." Louisa smiled at me. She laughed. "It's really good actually. It's all in there, I can't think that there is anything else left. You have opened yourself up as wide as you can, there are no secrets in this process, and you have been honest to a fault, and the tests and reports are all back. You are ready to submit."

"Really? We are done. Ready to submit?" Henri stopped pacing, came over and scooped me out the chair, hugged me and started to dance to the music in his head. I felt light as a feather, all the stress of it falling away.

"Aw, you two, give over! Put her down Henri! Training is done, interviews complete and now so is the form. I will submit this today! Now, it is 8.25am and you should open that door!"

With that Henri twirled me one last time, put me down, looked into my eyes and said, "Our new chapter starts now." With that he unbolted the door, opened it, and let in the morning sunshine and the hum of people rushing by to get to work. He turned back to us, "See it's a failure!" before laughing hard at his Bottom joke.

"Hello mate, any chance of a trim?" Our first customer walked in, and just like that our shop began its new life as a barbers.

Lupi By Name, Loopy By Nature

July passed by in a blur as busy life stuff took hold as we were fully occupied with both the opening of our new shop and we had now decided to sell our old shop business, so the glowy satisfaction of submitting our application form had now fallen away. Our new shop was ramping up with new customers as each day passed and we had already needed to recruit a new barber to help. I was now upstairs decorating the rooms we had plans for in order to follow through on the goal of bringing in more income, so me taking a year off work would make life a little easier for us. We had decided we were going to let the four rooms out to health practitioners: chiropractors, therapists, reflexologists, acupuncturists, that kind of thing. Two of the four rooms were decorated and ready for the therapists, and I had just started work on the third.

Sundays were the best days though; Henri wasn't working, and we got the chance to slow down and do nothing but be us. Just after we opened the shop, our first Sunday rolled round; we took a long hot walk through the dusty, dry fields parched by the scorching sun; summer had really delivered this year. We stepped into the cool relief of the woods, making our way down to the stream. Whilst Digby was splashing about in the water to cool off, we sat on the grassy bank, shoes off and feet dipped in, playfully splashing each other as we did so, I mused, "I wonder where we will be this time next year."

"We will have our family then, I am sure of it, and we will be planning a summer of fun, maybe the three of us and Digby can go on a road trip. Drive to the Lake District or across to France in a camper van. Adventure and the fun stuff in life!"

I smile at the thought of it, the perfection of it.

....

At around the same time that day, cars arrived at the top of a hill in the middle of a small English village. Police and social workers climbed out of their hot, stuffy cars and gathered together, ready to descend on a nearby flat to arrest a man and woman and take their children into the care of the local authority under police protection.

A few days earlier, it was noted by social workers that the parents of five children had failed to turn up to planned immunisations for their eleven-month-old twins without informing either the surgery or their allocated social worker. They were already firmly in the sights of the social team as seven years, earlier, the father was arrested for assaulting his wife whilst she was pregnant. The list of misdemeanours was plentiful both before this incident and afterwards.

The non-attendance in an important immunisation appointment meant a relook at their file and in that month alone, the father had breached his court order meaning the bailiff had applied for an eviction warrant request. In addition to this he was recorded flying a very noisy remote-control helicopter out in the communal garden at nearly midnight, smoking cannabis in the communal corridors and peering into the downstairs windows of the neighbour's son's bedroom, shouting and frightening both the neighbour's son and his wife.

Five days before the removal of the children, a legal meeting convened to discuss the increasing concerns regarding the neglect of the children and the looming eviction notice. Plans were put into motion to organise emergency accommodation for the children.

Two days after this meeting, the mother gave birth to a baby that no one knew she was due to have, including her doctor, so she could continue to take illicit drugs that she had come to depend on. The baby was airlifted to hospital as the baby's life hung in the balance. Post-birth, the baby tested positive for amphetamines in its system. This drug test, in turn, prompted an out-of-hours social working team to visit the father and the five children who were solely in his care that night. It was noted that the flat was extremely dirty, and the children subdued.

The day after that, the mother came home without her newborn baby, which takes us up to date with the police and social workers readying themselves to raid the flat the following morning.

They didn't need to bust down the door; the parents complied with the requests of the social workers and police officers. What the social workers found in the flat was blatant neglect, staring at them in the face. The flat itself was filthy; faeces behind the sofa, rubbish littered all over the floor, overflowing ashtrays, evidence of drug paraphernalia and drugs too. The children, all under the age of seven years old, were scooped up by the social working team. The twins were found in a cot amongst cans of cola, lager, and crisp packets. They, too, were filthy, covered in their own faeces with dirt wedged in the creases of their skin. They were not plump, gurgling, contented babies but quiet, resigned, skinny babies. The social workers lifted them out of their cots, down the cold concrete stairwell, out into the fresh air and into clean car seats. The social workers leave with the children and Jane and Andrew are left to the police for questioning. A few miles away, the eldest child was taken, confused and scared from his primary school by the social working team.

The twins were taken miles from this village to an emergency foster home by the sea. The fosterer, Mary, opened her door, ready to take in her new foster children and took a step back when she saw them. They smelt bad. "I thought the chap in the office said they were eleven months old; these babies can only be five months old, right? My goodness, they are filthy, grey with grime and scum." The social worker fills Mary in on as much background as is relevant to their brief stay with her. They have no belongings; there is nothing to hand over. Mary bathes them and dresses them in clean clothes from her extras box she keeps for emergency's. She feeds their tiny bodies and rocks them to sleep.

The social worker goes home and throws her own clothes in the bin; they are soaked in dirt. She decides she would rather not wear them again anyway; they would only remind her of the worst place she has been to in a long time.

....

July was coming to an end, and we wondered if we had a Panel date set yet, so I put in a call to Louisa. "Gosh guys no not yet! The department is snowed. They will get to it; I'll see if I can push it to the top of the pile! I will be in touch."

So, on we went, running the businesses, walking Digby, seeing friends, painting, and decorating the rooms upstairs. Summer was in full swing; the fields were parched and yellow now from the intense heat, summer flowers drooped full of pollen, ready for the hustle of the bees, and there were regular trips to the sea for swimming and plenty of ice creams.

One Tuesday night, I was preparing a dinner of roast chicken and mashed potatoes when the phone rang out, it was Louisa. "Hey! You guys ok? I have news. Can I come and see you tomorrow?"

"Yes, yes of course. Is it good news? Have they looked at the application form?"

"Let's chat tomorrow, lots to tell you. Ten o'clock?"

As I put down the phone, my old pal anxiety creeps back into my chest. I have not felt this feeling for a while. *Louisa didn't reassure me, that is why I am feeling this tightness, something is off, I am sure of it.*

The door slams downstairs. Henri. I get to the top of the stairs before he does and start this dance, where I shift from foot to foot. "What's happened babe?"

"Well," I start before the words just tumble out, "Louisa called, and she needs to see us tomorrow, she won't say why.

I think it is bad news. I feel it might be. Am I paranoid? What do you think?"

"I think you need to chill out, what can be wrong? I am starving and exhausted, it was busy today. Our shop is going to need more barbers soon, but I don't want to think about that now, I want to take a cold shower, eat some of the delicious food that I can smell and snuggle on the sofa watching that end of that drama from last night. Let's just chill." I nod trying to push the niggling, uncomfortable feelings aside.

I slept fitfully most of that night rolling around my fears, by around 4am I gave up on sleep opting for trashy reality TV with endless cups of Earl Grey tea for comfort, by the time Henri woke at 6.30am I was exhausted and impatient for ten o'clock to arrive.

I stood under a lukewarm shower for a long time enjoying the noise of it drowning out my inner thoughts, washing away the anxiety and soothing sore, tired eyes.

Louisa buzzed the doorbell on the dot of ten o'clock, Henri went down, and I clicked the kettle on to boil, setting out our mugs for tea. I could hear low mummering voices downstairs at the door, I finished making the tea and called down to them, what was taking so long?

Settled on the sofa, both of us stared at her expectantly.

"Look, I'm going to cut straight to it." *I knew it.* "The application is good, mostly it has passed through, there is a huge 'but' coming. I am sorry and I want you to know I wholeheartedly disagree, but they will not take the application any further unless ..."

Impatiently I cut in, "Sorry what? They are terminating our application?"

"Not as such if you agree to what they are asking for. I am sorry but Loretta, there is no easy way to say this, they have deemed you too unstable to adopt. I do not agree, I must make this clear to you guys." *Unstable. Can't adopt, too unstable to be a mother.*

I do not know what to say, rendered speechless I just stare at my feet. Henri speaks, "This is absolutely crazy; what do they mean? Why?" He steals a look at me and his face is full of confusion and concern.

"I am so sorry. Loretta on the form you admitted you were in therapy, and we all know it has been marvellous for you, but it does not fit their tick boxes. At the risk of sounding twee, you are the square peg trying to squeeze into their small round hole."

I feel like I've been punched in the stomach, but I find my voice. "Right, so, they ask us to be honest, so I completely open up to the process, told them I was there to be the best version of myself for adoption, for a child and you are saying it has gone against me? They just think I am mental now do they?" My voice is on the edge of breaking. "Who are these people?" My voice now becoming louder, screechier. I pause, "It's Doreen, isn't it? She has always had a kind of beef with me."

"She is just one of the leads on this application assessment. It is not all her decision. I promise she is not as bad as you think she is. It does not mean the end."

"How can it not mean the end? I am unstable apparently. Unable to mother. Christ. Henri I am so sorry." I turn to him and as I do, he pulls me into a bear hug and here come the tears I have been trying so hard not to shed. I chastise myself for always bloody crying.

"Loretta, if it's any consolation, I think you would be the best kind of mother. We need to fight this, and we can. I need access to Pru. She needs to submit a report stating that you are not an angry person or grieving still or replacing what you have lost. Will you ask her if I can phone her, yes?"

"That's all I have to do to get back on track?"

"Not exactly. They want you to submit yourself to a three-hour psych evaluation." Louisa almost whispered the last bit.

"A what?" Henri was even more incensed now. "Why should she, she is not insane?" *'She' is right here.*

"No but it is the only way to get you back on track, without it, they will not consider your application. I'm so sorry. It can be done here in your home; in fact, they would rather do it here as you will be more relaxed."

I sniffed and wiped my eyes and nose with my sleeve, always keeping it classy. "Yes. Yes. I'll do it. Set it up." My mind is made up instantly; I've come this far. What's one more humiliation to add to the list?

Louisa left after half an hour of reassurance to remember they do not know me, that it is not the end, that I should try and not take it to heart.

The rest of the morning was just a series of tasks. My mind shut down and I could only concentrate on what I needed to do. *Do not think about it. Keep moving forward. One step, then another.* I called Pru and left a message asking for an extra session as soon as possible. Pulled on my painting clothes for the shop. Drank a coffee, staring out the window at the Abbey, marvelling at its magnificent presence, how deep its foundations must be, how much adversity it must have endured, and its strength. I need some of that. I put together a salad tapas lunch for us both, clipped Digby to his lead and walked up the high street to the shop, my head held as high as I could muster. *Keep smiling.*

My job today was to gloss the window frames in room four. I thrust up the dusty paint-chipped sash window and the hubbub of the high street floated in, filling the room with sound over my own negative internal chatter, people going about their business, the chimes of the Abbey ring out telling me it is midday as I started to sand down the old window frames.

No one knows. Everyone is oblivious, I am going to break again, I can feel the spiral in my mind. My body could not give us children and now my mind is following suit. Unstable. I prize open the lid of the glossy white paint and dip my paintbrush in. Its gloppy consistency drips from the brush. I start to paint dripping globules of sticky white paint over the dust sheets as I go. I don't care.

What a complete loser you are. How can you do this to Henri? I did everything they asked of me. It's my fault, I failed again. The tears teetered at the back of my eyes, I squeezed them tight to stop them coming, shaking my head. *Do not feel sorry for yourself, you did this, you are unstable and more bloody crying just proves they are right.*

"Hello you!" I freeze, brush dripping more gloss everywhere. Zena. I forget we had a meeting in all of this goopy mess today. I turned and force a smile, "Goodness hello, I am so sorry I forgot we were meeting. I've had a morning of it." She smiles then throws her head back and laughs and when she refocuses on me, a single rebel tear has broken free and is running down my cheek.

"Oh, my goodness what is wrong?" Zena is kind to her core, and I have known her a while. I am in her team for a skincare brand I sell, she is no longer just a team leader to me but a friend, someone I both admire and respect. She has no children by choice, but that does not stop her understanding my need for a family. I can't answer her, I just start sobbing as soon as I open my mouth to speak. Zena steps forward and gets to her knees as if I am a child that needs someone to stoop to my level to console me. She gives me a big hug which brings forth hysteria, uncontrollable silent wailing. Somewhere deep inside me I am ashamed, but I cannot stop the sadness and pain from tumbling out. I try and explain between gulping in air. Words get swallowed and I am not making any sense. Some twenty minutes later, I finally started to calm down. I attempt a new explanation.

"They called me unstable; I know I look it right now breaking like this, but it's knocked me. Unstable Zena, to be a mother, not mother material. Our very last chance and I have stuffed it up again. My body is broken and now my mind has followed into the pit of despair."

Zena is suitably appalled for me; she is angry and sad. She soothes and holds my hand. We have tea, we talk some more before she needs to leave. I apologise for being such a mess. She leaves and we have not even spoken about skincare.

Henri replaces Zena's kindness with his own, reassuring me it will be ok; he thinks that if anyone can get through the psych test it is me. He gently suggests I go home to rest and snuggle into Digby's fur despite the heat, maybe succumb to sleep. Outside, the day has changed, it is raining, but I walk home in sunglasses anyway.

....

The twins spent only seven days in Mary's care, with other children coming and going as their new placements became available to them.

The social workers have reconvened and started care proceedings by creating a care plan for them. An interim care order has been granted by the court, the twins will be split from their siblings and placed with a foster family in the private foster agency sector. The two middle siblings have formed close bonds, so they need to stay together, and the oldest one needs to reduce his stress and anxiety after looking after his younger siblings in such adversity. The twins will be joined by their newborn sibling as soon as the doctors say the baby is medically fit for discharge from hospital. The birth parents will be allowed to have supervised contact twice weekly.

It had been noted in each of the siblings' files that there had been an increasingly high level of concern with each of the children's physical and emotional wellbeing since the birth of the twins. Consistently failing to meet the children's basic food and shelter needs, the children's safety and emotional wellbeing compromised, failing to ensure the children are clean and presentable in appearance causing potential stigmatisation. The birth parents' use of street drugs severely impaired their ability to protect and care for their children, reflecting deeply misplaced priorities. Their addiction led to financial neglect, as they failed to pay rent and relied on emergency food parcels to survive. Furthermore, the drugs likely diminished the effectiveness of the birth father's psychiatric medication, heightening the risk of domestic violence within the household. This cycle of substance abuse and instability created an unsafe and neglectful environment for the children.

The care team had found a foster home where they believed the twins would have their physical needs met, where they will start to develop strong identities, a safe, stable, and stimulating environment where their development is unimpaired by the failure to meet their basic needs.

Jojo waited for her new foster children to arrive and in preparation for their arrival, had bought some new toys to add to the ones already there. She had one of everything but needed to double up. With four days' notice, she managed to get a car seat, double buggy, second cot, fresh pyjamas, and new cot duvets, one in pink with mice on it and the other with a Thomas the Tank Engine design. Jojo did not know that the twins were coming with no belongings of their own, only what Mary had managed to buy for them in the last seven days packed into a plastic tub.

Jojo had not long had her last foster child adopted after two years of living with her. The little girl had arrived at three days old and stayed until she was nearly two. Her heart was broken, but her job was done, and she had spent eight months with no foster children in her home, so she had time to grieve her goodbye. Jojo knew it was time. She was ready for new children to mend her heart. Jojo is a sassy and striking blonde; in her heart, she is full of love and joy, her life is full of laughter. She laughs loud and hard, knowing that humour pulls her through some of the trauma she has witnessed. She brings a sense of fun to her foster children as well as showing them right from wrong, tackling the night terrors, the bad learned behaviour. She will always side with her foster children; she is in their corner. Children trust her.

Already at home were her husband Rick, her two teenagers, Joel and Steph, a Turner and Hooch breed of dog called Wilma and an angry twenty-one-year-old parrot called Spooky. Her four-bedroom home is clean and cosy; the hallway runs into the living room, which is long. Along one wall is the sofa and a sleeping cot and along the other is the fireplace and huge wall-mounted TV. Alongside that is the computer table. The room leads to the dining room and open-style kitchen. Two patio sliding doors give way to a glimpse of a lush green, well-tended garden. All this is a bright contrast to the dark, messy, and filthy flat the twins had become accustomed to in the short eleven months living with their birth parents.

They arrived with Mary, their own social worker, and a huge amount of paperwork. Whilst the social worker got busy on a risk assessment of her home, Mary handed over the twins and the little information, she knew about them. Jojo listened to how the twins arrived with her filthy faeces behind their ears, in their hair, how they were dark grey with dirt and the nappy rash that was so awful thanks to soiled nappies not being changed even on a daily basis.

Despite being eleven months old, the twins were in clothes for six-month-old babies; the boy twin was especially thin; his head was huge, but his body was thin and narrow. His dark brown almond-shaped eyes sunken into his eye sockets. They were both very quiet and sat very still staring at the toys, having not ever laid eyes on so much colourful joy. Jojo opened her arms and her heart to the twins and they both tumbled into a new world full of love and nurture.

....

Pru waited at the door to her office wearing a smile and a summery yellow and green strappy dress. I stepped into her sun-filled room and embraced the familiar smell and the colours, letting them soothe me a little. I dropped my keys and water bottle at my feet and sank into the low-slung chair. Pru, as is customary for our sessions, waited until I spoke. I looked at her, then at my feet and instead of a steady stream of tears threatening to fall, a rising had begun to climb in my chest, a tenseness in my shoulders before a tirade of words fired out at her. An angry muddle of sentences as I explained last week's events in all their grave details.

Pru sat very still. "This obviously has made you very angry."

"Pru, that is stating the bloody obvious, isn't it? Wouldn't you be?"

"We are not talking about me."

Is she for real? I was angry and she was making me angrier. I was not ready to calm down.

"Ok, well yes, I am angry, I am absolutely furious, no scrub that, I am livid. How dare they just make up their minds on whether I am capable or not capable of mothering a child. Stable or unstable. Am I unstable?"

"What do you think? Are you unstable? Tell me." I wanted to yell louder, is she provoking me, poking at the bear inside me because it was awake already.

"Right now, this very bloody minute, yes." An omission. I had confessed. I pause for breath and possibly clarity, then I realise my rant has come to an end. The red mist is receding, my anger subsiding and falling to where my keys and water bottle lay.

"First of all, this is not how you should be acting in the face of adversity, this anger you are holding onto will literally get you nowhere. Ask yourself, be truthful, is this about something else?"

I have learnt to become comfortable with the uncomfortable silences between our conversations, so I take my time to think, bring my breath under control, pull my shoulders down, sit back into the chair.

"What makes you unstable right now in this moment?" She presses me for an answer. I sigh audibly, knowing that until Pru gets an honest answer, she will not stop with this line of questioning. There is no hiding from Pru.

"I guess I went to a place where I wasn't thinking straight; I was thinking more with my pain, pain from the past and pain that my future may not be what I am currently fighting so hard for. I am fearful of it. I was being hostile, even to you and I trust you. Don't worry you are not the only one, Henri got it with both barrels too. I wanted to hurt with my words, I guess, because I feel so much hurt."

Pru crosses her legs, tucking her skirt under them as she does so and shifts in her chair before she speaks again. "My concern is not that you cannot mother but more about what happens if this kind of anger gets in the way of mothering. In the future, say you have your child and if you feel this kind of pain, this type of red-hot anger, how does that play out? You do not know this yet, but children have an uncanny way of pushing buttons and boundaries you did not know you had."

I am not sure what to say, this is the second punch in my stomach in a week. I feel a bit sick. How could I possibly ever feel this kind of anger towards a child, that would make me no worse that the adults that had failed them in the first place. I whisper, "Would you say I am out of control?"

"No. Mostly no. Do I think you are unstable? Actually, no if I must answer that. We all find anger inside ourselves. It is how we direct it that counts. What I believe is, no matter what has been said in this room, as that is done in the strictest of confidence, I will say you have worked hard, and you have birthed a new version of you, are they wrong? Well, I would say yes, but like I said I can only deal with the facts."

"Will you speak with them? They want to hear from you."

"I will need written consent from you to allow me to talk to them. I can only give them facts, I can not and will not comment on whether I think you will make a good mother. What I *think* bears no relevance. You understand?"

"Yes." I lean forward, putting my elbows on my knees and my hands over my face and I silently weep, exhaustion washing over me. "I am so tired Pru. Tired of all the tears, of being under the microscope. Tired of fighting."

"Remember what you are fighting for. You are much stronger than you know. You will win this."

....

After introducing the twins to the fun of toys and playtime, and as gently as she could, Jojo changed endless nappies as much as she needed to in order to treat possibly the worst nappy rash she had ever seen, in both the twins. Jojo cooked an early tea of fish fingers, chips, and baked beans, nothing fussy. A teatime that was soft and comforting, something they could explore with their fingers. Possibly their first time in highchairs, she will never know for sure, but she observed the boy twin stuffing the food into his mouth as if he had never seen a full plate of food before. He ate quickly, every morsel on his plate, hoovered up, Jojo felt in her gut that she was literally feeding a starving child. He rewarded her with a big, beaming, mucky smile, the baked bean juice dripping off his chin and smeared across his face. Jojo returned his smile knowing for the first time his tummy was full.

Bath time was nothing but upsetting. Both the twins took one look at the bath and screamed and yelled indicating something quite awful had happened around water. So, she drew a very shallow bath for a quick splash around with plastic ducks and bubbles both in the bath and blowing ones into the air to distract them. She never strayed from their side and her daughter had joined her to help too. She marvelled at her daughter, still in school but with such a natural ability with children, so calm and giving them all the fun with her warm laughter. The twins were all cosy in their new pyjamas, so both her and Steph bottle-fed the twins warm milk to induce sleepiness whilst watching In The Night Garden and gently rocking them in their arms.

That night's sleep was very broken for most of the house with the twins waking regularly and not just crying on waking but waking with alarming shrieking. Night terror is very common for children that come to her. She nursed them through as best she could until the daylight slipped under the curtains, and they slept soundly again.

Jojo knows she has to run to the timetable that is set for her by the twins' social workers, but it did not stop her from disagreeing with being asked to take the twins to a contact centre the day after they had arrived. They had barely settled in, and today, they had to go and see the birth parents, under close supervision of course. At contact, they would see their siblings again too, that was one blessing. She comforted her tired self, knowing that at least she would be there for the twins when they came out.

She drove them to the centre of a nearby town, dutifully getting there on time. The first thing she noticed when she handed over the twins was that the birth mother had no teeth as she introduced herself, taking the little girl from Jojo awkwardly into her arms. She told Jojo it was a calcium deficiency, but Jojo suspected it had to do with rubbing too much amphetamine on her gums. She had seen it all before and was too long in the tooth for the excuses. Contact went pretty much without a hitch; the twins appeared happy enough and the birth parents were, at the very least, polite. From the outside looking in, it would appear that nothing much was wrong.

··········

The morning of the psych evaluation had arrived and as to be expected the anxiety monkey was rampaging through my body, restricting my breath, and gifting me with the worst headache. I longed for a good night's sleep again and to shut down the constant internal negative vitriolic chatter. I couldn't eat breakfast as I felt too nauseous so I mainlined coffee instead to keep me alert.

The doorbell chimed, announcing Dr Margot Turner had arrived. As much as I was a jellified mess inside, I steadied myself and plastered on just the right amount of smile but also giving away a hint of worry about our session together. First impressions and all that jazz. This was an extremely important hurdle to jump over, or it all ended here, today. *No pressure Loretta.*

Dr Margot was a short, thin woman with tiny shoulders, too tiny to be carrying the enormous bag she lugged in for her stature. Her nut-brown coloured eyes matched her shoes and the oversized leather bag. She wore jeans and a flowery printed shirt. Plain gold earrings in her ears and soft make-up in direct contrast to her very severe pixie hairstyle. She looked wise, there was an air of knowingness about her. I invited her in and offered coffee. I poured myself a tall glass of water, the large caffeine intake this morning had started to take hold judging by the juddering in my veins, or was that just jangly nerves?

We settled on opposite sofas in the light living room, there will be no hiding in the shadows. She was gentle when she spoke as if she knew I may break apart at any moment. She thinks I am unstable, that is what they have told her.

We began.

"Ok Loretta let's get going. It is a long session, but I must tell you first that whilst I have read their conclusions and your application form, I am currently sitting here completely impartial. I am an independent psychologist." I nod. "You know the drill I am guessing from your own therapy sessions so, let's start by asking you why you wish to adopt a child."

I felt like I had accidentally put my hand up to ask a question in a conference, all eyes on me.

Would I offer anything inciteful? Can I convince her I am a good person with a big heart, someone ready to bring in a child and mother them? I remembered what Henri told me this morning, *just be yourself, that is all that matters*. Digby was lying on my feet, he lifted his head and looked at me. I cleared my throat. "It's simple really, I have so much love inside me, inside both of us and there are so many children without love in their lives. Bringing a child into our family will give us the opportunity to change a child's life. We have a lot of love to give."

"How? How can you change a child's life?"

"Well, I am part of a loving Italian family, so they will always have people around them who will love them from all angles. My sister has so much to give too, she will be there always. Henri's family is wonderful too and there are no grandchildren yet so it would mean a lot to them, they are so generous and giving and will spoil them in all the right ways. Then there is the other side of things, I speak Italian so I can bring them up bilingually, as we are self-employed, I am able to be free to take off as much time as needed to ensure attachment and nurturing."

"I see. So, lots of people willing to give. Uh-huh." She pauses, looking down at her notes. *Why is she not writing this down?*

"These are all ideal answers, run of the mill, saying what you think I need to hear. I need to drill down a little bit more, I need to find you. Why are you in therapy?"

I need to be me. I need to answer as me not the version of me I've perfected for training or in front of social workers. I take a deep breath.

"The truth is I was broken that's why. I was incapable of loving myself, let alone anyone else. When my body failed me, I became unlovable. I didn't love me. I made myself unlovable. I was snappy and sharp. I disengaged from the world. No one truly understood. No one really tried to understand. Henri, yes, but not my family or my closest friends. No one wanted to hear my answers, feel my pain, hear me wailing." My voice had gone up a few octaves, Digby felt it and had sat up placing his head on my lap. My golden boy then jumped onto the sofa and settled beside me, his head back on my lap, nudging my hands. I bent and kissed the top of his soft, furry head and rested my arm around him, pulling him closer. "I needed help. Being a woman who wasn't able to perform, do, as a woman should disabled me. I've always longed for children; it was always part of my life plan."

"We are getting somewhere now; can you add to that?"

"We always wanted to adopt, but we couldn't do both, as in IVF and adoption together, at the same time, so given our ages, we plumped for IVF first. It never occurred to me it wouldn't happen. It derailed me, sent me off course."

"What were your biggest fears?"

"That's hard to answer, but mostly losing Henri. He is my rock; we are so strong together. Look how far we have come. We talked about it, and I told him he could leave me, leave us, and I would understand."

"Did you mean it?" Dr Margot was becoming more conversational, almost like she was invested in my story now. *Still not writing anything down.*

"Yes, you know I really did. I thought little of myself, a loser, a dropout. Why would he be with me? I could not give him children. Obviously, you know that he stayed, but more than that, he showed me true love and commitment. Worked harder to afford therapy for me, to help me heal. I walked through the door to therapy because I was shown such love from him, I felt the same way towards him. I did it initially for him, but soon that gave way to me realising I was worth it and then I did it for me. The dark thoughts did not deserve a place inside that love. Pru showed me how I could let go of the failure, the pain, and the anxiety." I pulled Digby even closer, and he rolled onto his back for a belly rub.

"True love is a wonderful joy. Why do you feel the social working team think you are unstable?"

"I am an easy target. I do not fit the mould, their mould. I am expressive, opinionated, and real. I am also nervous and anxious and cover that with ill-timed jokes. I do not tick the boxes. I'll be honest here; I was unstable. When I first walked into Pru's office, I was so unstable I wasn't even sure I wanted to live. Now though, now, that is an insult to Henri, Digby, and myself. It hurts to think that's the perception of my mental health. I have worked tirelessly on myself. It's been dark, and I have had to face so many demons, but I am here feeling the best I have felt since, well, since we started IVF. I am coming back to myself, and it feels good. I am not an unstable person. Not anymore."

"Would you say that you would be able to handle the many ups and downs that motherhood can throw at you?"

"How do I know? I cannot promise anything except to always pledge that I will try my best. How can anyone know? I can back myself, but only I know that I walk the path of someone who has built a new life, a life with a wider lens. I am gentler with myself, and I would like to think that as a mother, I would be able to use these new skills to survive parenting too."

Silence. O bollocks, I've been too me. Too honest. O well, I'm going all in now.

"This process has opened us up in more ways than we expected. We have laid ourselves bare. I am here completely naked in the sense that there are no secrets. Parents that conceive naturally become mothers and fathers; can they say the same? Do they go through a process similar to this? No.

Don't get me wrong I understand why we are tested this way, the children can not go through anymore trauma but still, it is invasive and raw." Digby yawns loudly. He's bored, heard it all before and ready for a walk around the park.

Dr Margot asks more questions, less about me and more about our environment, religion, how I would deal with tantrums, that kind of thing. She then asks for some water. Returning from the kitchen, she says, "Ok, let's start again. Why do you want to adopt?"

We go through the same questions again, sometimes worded slightly differently but mostly exactly the same another three times. That is why she writes nothing down and by the fourth round of questioning, she knows me and my story pit pat. During the questioning, we had some more coffee, ate some biscuits, thrown open the windows to circulate air. Digby has given up his vigil, sensing I am now relaxed and goes to sleep in the hallway where it is cool and quiet.

Dr Margot announces we are done. I fall back onto the sofa and breath out audibly. She swaps from interviewer mode to friendly mode. "You survived it! How was that?"

"Brutal!" I joke "Ok I guess, long and hot and I think my voice is wearing out!"

"You did great."

"I did?" My eyes widen and I shift to the edge of the sofa. "Can I ask, did I pass the test?"

She smiles. "You did. I shouldn't say this as it should just go into my report, but I can see it means so much to you. You didn't just pass, you have demonstrated that you are not only stable as a person, in fact as a mother should be, but you have shown me such strength and courage that in my opinion, for what it is worth you and Henri, in fact, have the ability to adopt siblings. Yes, completely stable. I will be recommending that."

"Gosh, I don't know what to say. Thank you. Thank you so much."

We exchanged goodbyes and I rush to find my phone. Six missed calls from Henri and one from Louisa. I lie on the floor next to Digby and whisper, "We did it boy, we passed the test. I passed. I love you." I bury my face in his fur and this time cry big happy tears before I call Henri.

The Panel

The horror stories for the Panel that we had heard whilst in adoption training over the year were enough to put the frighteners on the hardiest of couples. Louisa was completely honest with us and told us that a yes or no from the adoption Panel is final; their decision is what will take us forward, or not. We know that up to fourteen people could be sat in front of us with our application form at their fingertips and a list of their own questions. It was going to be a pressurised environment to be in. This kind of scrutiny reminded me of school trips to Bath to perform in the drama festival on stage in front of the other competitors and that judging Panel. The reminder made me green with nerves.

We were scheduled to sit in front of the Panel in late August, but the question over my mental health being too unstable to be a parent set us back a few months. Now that my emotional resilience had been proven to be strong, thanks to the glowing report submitted by the rather wonderful, (as I refer to her now,) Dr Margot we had finally received a date of 14th October.

The rest of the hot summer was spent working in our shop, slowly and steadily building a successful and popular business up. Long workdays but we were crammed with new and returning customers, new ideas, launching the rooms upstairs, endless admin. We were so busy in the barber side of the shop we had taken on a part-time member of staff and were searching for another full-timer to join the expanding team too now that we knew the earning potential was there for them. Plans were afoot to add in some retail for men like styling products and shampoos and Henri had started designing our own clothing brand too. Our down time was mainly spent coastal with Digby at our side. The coast held space for us to just be, helping us to breathe easier, bask in the sun on our skin, bathe in the cool English sea, walk the pathways, and chat, nothing seemed to pressure us there. Digby loved it too, he loved to race to the water's edge before ducking his head under the water and swim out, he delighted all around him as he swam under the salty water, retrieving stones for us to throw for him before getting out and rolling in the sand.

I also said goodbye to Pru. Sound the trumpets, I had graduated from therapy and was navigating life completely on my own again. Our last session was a little like our first, with many tears from me, but these tears had been transformed into those of happiness and gratitude. To my surprise, before I left my sessions, Pru thanked me, saying she had learnt some big lessons from me in resilience. She praised my ability to prise myself open and accept the process and my reward was that I was stronger, more independent in a way that I could now count on myself, and I knew who I was and what I stood for. I feel I should have left with a medal and a certificate for all the work I had done but I settled for walking taller through the rest of my life. Her door, she said was always open if I needed to come back.

The morning we were meeting with the Panel, we woke earlier than normal. We walked Digby across the white frost-covered fields, we could see our breath in the air, we were wrapped up in big coats and had donned wellies that crunched with each step we took, the ground underfoot being frozen solid. We didn't talk much, each of us in our own head taking in the beauty of the winter-filled fields, breathing out cool white plumes from our lungs, the sun a yellow haze behind the thick clouds that hung over our heads, hand in hand as we walked.

The night before we talked about what to wear. I said we should probably wear suits or something formal. Henri laughed, "It's not court, we need to be ourselves, when the hell have you ever known me to wear a suit? Wedding day the exception. I think it is more important to be comfortable, don't you? It's going to be bloody awful enough let's face it."

He was right. So, he wore jeans and a T-shirt, and I wore leggings, a simply smock dress with minimal make-up so if the tears fell as freely as they had the last few years at least I wouldn't have streaks of make-up coursing down my face. We left a lot earlier than we needed to and arrived in the car park where it all started just over one year ago. The building looked the same. Nothing about the building had changed, but we were forever changed. We were forever changed by this process. The Pollyanna optimism fallen and our eyes fully open with what happens and has happened to children living in the care system, how that system is flawed but still safer than what came before. Now, our journey to adoption will be finalised here today.

We climbed out of our newly purchased family-sized car. I turn to Henri and lean into him, "I am ready. I don't think we could have done anymore and now I am ready for this." He smiles. "Me too."

"I mean I think I might be sick with nerves but let's get this over with."

We walk into the building and wait at the little hatch window that is already wedged open. From across the office, we hear the receptionist. "Hang on, I am on my way over, understaffed today." She huffed and sighed loudly as she padded across the office to the hatch. "Right then, who are you?"

"Loretta and Henri Lupi-Lawrence here for the Panel process."

"Lupi what now?"

"Lawrence."

"Oh I can't see you."

Alarm coursed through my already charged body. Henri laughed and turned away adding, "You can't make this shit up."

"Ahhh got you. Sit down and wait to be called."

We found seats, Henri still chortling, "Bet she went to charm school!" I grinned back despite myself.

After a twenty-minute wait, a breathless Louisa ran down the stairs, "Sorry we are running behind, but everyone is here now. How are you feeling? Silly question, don't answer that. You are going to ace it. Let's go through to the prep room."

She led us down a maze of corridors, through a series of heavy fire doors until we reached a small windowless room. A large table with some chairs tucked under it, a water cooler standing on top of a small unit. Nothing on the off-white textured wallpapered walls. "Right, coffee?"

We declined. "So, today's Panel is ten. Doreen and two of her top tier team members, a GP, Ben who you met at one of the training sessions, I think, he's an adopter and another adopter you don't know. A counsellor, a psychologist and one of the heads of the local council. I am missing one. Anyway, they are all actually OK." I raised my eyebrows and as if reading my mind Louisa added, "Oh she will be fine; Doreen wants children to be adopted. She just has a funny way of showing it sometimes! I'll go and see if they are ready."

With that she left us alone. We looked at each other. Henri spoke first. "You've got this, we've got this."

I nodded, "We have." There was nothing more to say.

Louisa appeared once more. "It's time and you get to go in together. Sorry I can't come in with you, not allowed, but I will be waiting right here." She pointed to the door next to the room we were in. "Through there, good luck!"

I opened the door and together we shuffled in, once more propelled centre stage and our audience all looked up and stopped talking as we walked in. Ten pairs of eyes all turned to look at us. *Are we what they were expecting?* They were seated in a U formation, three on each side and four in the middle. Each of them had a glass of water and various hot beverages in mismatched china mugs and of course, each had a copy of our application form. The adoption experts. This is the same room we were in to learn what adoption was all about and then to learn about Foster to Adopt. I scanned the room from right to left whilst smiling and finding our chairs in front of the Panel. Henri squeezed my hand and then sat down. Doreen and her team to my right, and suited, more formal individuals to my left. A lady in a burgundy suit welcomed us in. She had the same colour lipstick on as her suit, older, dark greying hair that was wavy and landed on her shoulders. Glasses balanced on the end of her nose. Her voice felt silky. "Hello, do sit down, awful this isn't it? Must feel like you are an animal in a zoo, I am Marjory and I work at the council doing a host of boring but necessary jobs." She chuckled and the others loosened up a bit by joining in. *Hit the nail on the head there, Marjory.*

Doreen spoke. "This is Loretta and Henri, and you have their application in front of you should you need to refer to it. She turned to us. Let me introduce the Panel." Off she went around the room introducing people and I barely heard a word she said I was too busy picking Digby hair off my dark dress and forcing a big *please love us* smile onto my face. "We should kick off then Marjory."

"Yes, yes. Loretta, tell me what your relationship was like with your parents when you were younger and whether you will, adopt, so to speak, the same parenting style."

Here we go ...

So many questions came firing at us, how would you teach your children, how would you discipline them? What hobbies do you have? How long are your working hours? Will those hours change with children? Will you set boundaries for your children and what will they be? If they tantrum in a public place, how will you handle that? How are you prepared financially for adoption? Will you have a budget? Have you ever been through financial hardship? How did you cope? What makes you most afraid about adopting? Who is supporting you in this adoption process? Who will you count on? Do any of your family smoke? We answered all their questions, mostly taking it in turns. Does anyone around you have mental health issues? Do you have mental health issues?

"Loretta, I see you are in therapy. Tell me about that." The quiet lady in the plain blue suit spoke up.

"Well, I was broken and had become afraid of life, I guess, I hid in the shadows of life when I had always been out in front of it. I have always wanted children in my life, since I was a child, I dreamt of being a mother. I made plans for motherhood, then my body failed me when it came to it. I was miserable and I needed to fix myself before adopting because it is only right a child comes into a loving home not a sad one. I have done the work and now I know I am capable of being the best mother I can be to a child. I signed out of therapy at the end of the summer, and I am doing ok." I smile.

"But there were some concerns that you were unstable, surely that can become a reality again."

"Actually, I am going to step in here." Doreen interrupted. "Loretta willingly opened herself up to a psych evaluation and she has proven to be strong enough and emotionally stable so Karen, we can leave this line of questioning now I think, it is all in the report."

My eyes had moved over to rest on Doreen as she was speaking, and my mouth had involuntarily hung itself open in disbelief. *She has my back. Doreen has my back.* I smiled and looked down into my lap as questioning started again.

"Henri, we do not hear much about your parents across the application, can you tell us why?" Jane spoke, she was the psychologist in the room. She was elegant, sharply thin, and wearing loose clothing in cream and camel colours.

I looked at Henri expectantly and I see him shift uncomfortably in his chair not used to be being the one with the spotlight on him. "We live quite far away from them, but they are in my life of course. We all chat regularly."

"Are you not close? I get the feeling there is something there we are not seeing?"

Henri's face was screwed up in confusion. "Why? I mean why would you think that. They were interviewed did something come up there I don't know about?"

"I am concerned that they are not mentioned as part of the core support network."

I can see Henri struggling under the pressure of Jane's questioning. I jump in, "Henri's parents are wonderful salt of the earth people, but they live quite a bit away from us, and it wouldn't be fair to call on them at their age and expect them to come and help. They will one hundred per cent be in our child's life. Henri's mother is warm and interested in everything we introduce to them, and Henri's dad is wise, he's measured and so good-natured. They bring so much goodness to the table for a grandchild. Why wouldn't they be part of our core network, they are integral to our family dynamic, it just means we need to drive to them to see them, that's all."

"I see. Good. That's good." Henri breathes a long breath out and squeezes my thigh with gratitude.

Dr Rangeet speaks next. "Your medicals all look good, except I notice that Loretta, you are overweight. You mentioned earlier that you run and do yoga, but you still have an obese figure. Would you consider yourself healthy? In my opinion, I would think not. What do you intend to do to be in the best health for your child? You will be perhaps susceptible to heart problems and as we all know obesity is a problem in this country. You won't keep up with an energetic child."

Wow. He's talking to me as if I am the size of an elephant. It's true I am a bigger woman, but I am hardly enormous. I falter because his words have hurt me. "I am a size sixteen to eighteen and I do workout and I am doing my best to slim down. Dr Rangeet I went through eight years more or less of IVF and being poked, prodded, opened up, and injected with all kinds of drugs. I sport scars both inside and out and have physically lost parts of myself. I recognise that I am overweight, but my body has overcome so much, it's a wonder in fact. What my body has endured is incredible and it still takes me for runs, my heart still beats just as strong as yours does."

I falter, not sure I can go on Henri picks up the baton for me this time, "Also my wife is kind of perfect in every way and I do not for one minute accept this as a problem."

The room smiles, except Dr Rangeet who just nods and writes down some notes.

Doreen stands, "I think we are all done here. Thank you both of you, it's been a journey, eh?" She winks and sits down dunking a rich tea into what must be cold tea by now.

Marjory followed suit, wishing us well. We stood and left the room behind us to ruminate on our future.

We emerged from the room and Louisa was there as promised. "I listened in at the door, sounded good, well a bit of a grilling but you guys handled it. How do you feel?"

"Relieved it's done now." Henri moved into the little side room out of the corridor. I remained quiet, not sure how I was feeling. "When do we know? A few days or is it weeks?"

"Oh no, in the next twenty minutes or so."

What? Twenty minutes. I am not ready. Oh yes you are, it really is time. What if they reject us? What will we do?

"Loretta, are you OK you look pale?" Henri turned to look at me. "Babe?"

"Yup, I'm all good it's just this is a big deal and uh, soon we will know what the rest of our life will look like. Those ten people are discussing our future, they decide. It feels all a bit surreal."

We sat down and no sooner had we taken a seat, than Marjory popped her head around the door. I am pretty sure all three of us held our breath for a brief moment. "Let me put you out of your misery. You passed with flying colours. We think you will make amazing parents to a child or maybe children, we agree with Dr Margot that you should be considered for siblings. Congratulations." She smiled her burgundy smile. Louisa punched the air, Henri shouted 'yes' loudly and then started thanking Marjory profusely. He pushed his chair back and hugged me tight and then hugged Louisa too. I whispered to no one in particular, "We did it. We bloody did it!"

Eventually, back in the car park, we hugged for a while, and then our euphoria tipped over into an impromptu victory dance. We drove home in a daze, recalling parts of the questioning and planning an evening that included a bottle of Champagne, a fish and chip supper, with an added sausage for our furry boy.

....

Jojo was pleased. The twin boy was putting on weight. He had learnt how to run before he could walk, running at everything at high speed! He was always up for a game of something fun. He laughed all the time. He was looking healthier; that awful ridge-like line down his forehead where he was so thin had disappeared. The girl twin had definitely attached to her. Jojo had a new shadow, especially now the little girl had learnt to toddle around. She loved nothing more than to be picked up and cuddled. They had become part of the family and hearing them laugh was such a joy to Jojo, these little babies that once didn't know how to play or giggle.

Parties, Catalogues & Resumés

The first thing that happened after we passed the Panel was two weeks later, Louisa sent through resumes for two beautiful sisters, a three-year-old and a toddler of eighteen months. The girls were from Lambeth, London and needed a new home after being taken by social workers from their birth home after poverty had led the parents to despair and, ultimately, violence and crime. The children were both black. Their eyes were big and brown with tight curly hair, their childish beauty shining out through big, wide, toothy grins. Henri and I agreed we would like to meet them and move forward. No sooner had we made that decision that we got the call to say we had been turned down because we were living in a town that was too white. I can say with a degree of certainty that I didn't react very well to that decision. Since when did racism invade the lives of innocent children? Forever is the answer. I had been so naïve, and I was angry about it, for the children, for these little girls, the chance of a loving home and a good life snatched because we and our town were too white. After tons of reading about this topic, it turns out that transracial adoption is very much thought of as a second-best option and social workers would rather place black children in foster homes than have them adopted into a white family. Appalled but knowing we didn't have a say in white bureaucracy and that I had nowhere to go with my anger, I reluctantly dropped it, but I often wonder about the little girls from Lambeth.

In the third week past the Panel, profiles of homeless children came in thick and fast. All kinds of children, different ages, heights, blue eyes, green eyes, brown eyes, boys and girls, all staring down at the camera lens being photographed for our eyes in the hope of being adopted. Little synopses of their journeys in life so far. All hoping and wishing for their forever homes. Louisa told us we would know when the right child would come along.

A little blonde boy's profile landed in our email inbox. He was four years old with the bluest eyes I've ever seen and even blonder long hair. He was dressed in a fancy dress tiger outfit, but he wasn't grinning for the camera the way the little Lambeth girls had. His story was that he was born to a single mother in the northeast of the UK who struggled with mental health issues. She could not cope with him, as she hadn't been able to keep her first child, social services intervened once more. I could not pinpoint it, but I didn't think he was meant to be with us, and I lurched from feeling heartbroken that I had, in fact, just rejected a child to know that in my gut he was not the right child for us. I stared for a long time at that photo, and I kept coming back to it. Over and over, every time I looked at his picture, my stomach hurt. I felt sure he wasn't for us, but it was a feeling I was not at all happy with.

Next, we were sent catalogues. Catalogues of children, as if they were products from an Argos book, essentially shopping for a family. As we flipped the pages of children's eyes, all hoping they could catch our attention, they made me feel appalled at myself as we found ourselves saying no to brown eyes, as we both have blue eyes, no to the older kids no matter how cute they looked in the pictures, no to any child not white as we knew we lived somewhere too white so we would be turned down anyway. Ugh. "Is there no other way to do this?" I complained and set about moaning about the process for the hundredth time. It just all felt too icky. By the fourth catalogue we stopped even opening them as they came in.

We also got invited to adoption parties, something that we also found wasn't exactly tasteful. Invited to watch where children are playing, standing at the edge of a playground to observe whether there is a child there you like the look of. It's not unlike speed dating, as the kids whizzed by us playing with their friends. We felt like we were spying on the kids and that felt seedy somehow. Plus, with these parties, you were always eyeing up your competition, throwing side glances at other couples. Anxiety induced heaven.

Around the same time, my friend had just had her second baby, the same friend who had to cancel her skiing holiday the first time she was pregnant. I jumped on a train to London to help out with the new family dynamic over the first few weeks; now, her husband had gone back to work. One afternoon as we walked down the King's Road window shopping, we were chatting about the experience Henri and I had with the tail end of the adoption process, I explained about the little blonde boy and his profile.

"You know, what can you tell from a photo? I mean, what are you looking for? He's a little kid needing someone to love him, give him a home. Are you just scared you can't handle him? It's the same for all mums you know, we are all just feeling our way around parenting and trying to not to fuck it up. We do by the way; we all fuck it up a little."

Further along the road, as we peered into a baby shop window, I took out my phone as it started to ring, "Hey babe, you OK? Yeah, yeah, all good here, little Tara is wrapped up in a bundle of blankets and sleeping in her pram. Ooof you know, she looks like an angel. We are on King's Road. I've been thinking. Yes, hilarious dangerous I know! I think maybe we should go for it. With the little blonde boy. I mean, why not?"

Next, I put in a call to Louisa and left a message on her phone to call me about the little blonde boy. Louisa returned my call, "I think we will go for him. The little blonde boy. Is he still available to adopt?" I grimace as I ask, I feel like I am shopping.

"Well, yes, he is. Are you sure? What made you change your mind? You are sure, aren't you? Best thing to do is arrange a meet up and see how you feel after that." And that was that, our name was thrown into the ring for the little blonde boy.

Lucy and I went in search of a cafe to warm up with ~~bouee~~ fancy hot chocolates and some privacy so she could breastfeed her little Tara. Decision made. There was a small part of me that was still very unsure. Annoyed at myself for still feeling this way, I ordered not just a hot chocolate but a thick slice of indulgent chocolate cake with cream on the side. I told myself I was celebrating, but I was, in fact, finding comfort in cake, burying my uncomfortable feelings under lashings of sugar and cream.

....

The twins were content, putting on weight and mostly sleeping through the night. With it being so cold now, Jojo had bought the twins some new winter coats and some new toys to add to their new collection. Jojo had once more found her stride. She was about to take in the twins' baby sibling for a few weeks now that the doctors had rehabilitated the tiny baby from the enforced drug addiction during pregnancy to leave the hospital until the Foster to Adopt order came through.

She had just come off the phone from her agency boss requesting that she take some photos of the twins so that he could then, in turn, send them to the twins' social worker. The core social working team had decided all the children apart from the older one would be available to adopt. She enquired why not the oldest and was told he was considered too unsettled and that maybe at eight years old, he may be passed over for adoption anyway. She disagreed. Her heart felt sad and heavy for the twins' oldest brother, the one that had tried to keep them safe in the early days when he was so young himself.

The twins, fresh from an early afternoon bath after a particularly muddy session in the park earlier, were in their onesie pyjamas and playing with new toys by the patio windows. The light was bright this afternoon. She called them to the window to look at the squirrels and they tottered to her as if drunk, still not quite stable on their feet and put their hands on the glass to steady themselves. "Look at me!" They did and giggled at the same time. She clicked the button. JoJo was rather pleased. She had captured their chubby cheeks; one had blue eyes and mousey hair and the other had brown almond-shaped eyes with blonde hair. Both were looking bright-eyed and happy. Their cheeks were ruddy still from playing outside in the cold air then back home into a warm bath. Each twin had new tufts of hair growing on the top of their heads now too. The girl twin had a very cheeky look in her eye and JoJo knew she was about to do something mischievous that would make them both squeal with laughter. As soon as she lowered her phone from taking the picture, she did just that, she fell to her knees and crawled through her twins' legs, making him topple over and peals of laughter broke out from them both, filling the living room with life.

....

Louisa called us to say there was a hold-up with the little blonde boy as his birth mother had had a change of heart and was fighting the system, which was causing all kinds of problems as she prepared to fight for him in court and to add to that, she was also pregnant again. A reassessment needed to happen with his core social working team. In the meantime, would we want to see other profiles?

"Yes, do that, thanks Louisa. Can you keep us updated on his case as any news comes in?" I am not sure I sounded as upset as I should have been to hear that news plus, I was appalled at myself for having just called this child a 'case' and not by his name.

"Absolutely." Not sure Louisa sounded as convinced as she should have been to reassure me.

I stuck my arms into my winter coat and grabbed Digby's lead. Found my bag, stuffed it with homemade soups and rolls for our lunches and headed out to our shop. I needed some air. I was in no hurry to get to work. I took the long route round mulling over the last year. There was nothing post-Panel that was any easier than pre-Panel. It was just different. No prying eyes or forms or tests to pass but now we found ourselves in a long game of waiting, the children were waiting and so were we and somehow, we needed to move forward with our lives. Not pregnant but expecting a family, soon-ish.

Weeks later we had heard nothing from anyone, nothing of importance. I had convinced myself the next profile would be the one. Pinned all my hopes and dreams on it. The blonde boy had passed us by now. Our fates were not matched, which, let's face it, I knew anyway.

At the beginning of December, we got the email we had been waiting for. Longing for. An instantaneous connection to a picture of two beautiful grinning toddlers dressed in cosy onesies photographed at a window. Like raw wires meeting, a spark was lit and an engine roared. Memories fell in front of my eyes, the twins I was obsessed with in my class at school, how I marvelled at their closeness, their own language, their connection. Henri's medium session where his grandad came through with the words BOGOF. Twins. Being approved for sibling adoption. Every fibre of my body was alert. This, then, is what it was all for. Louisa was right; I did know when the right profile came along. These innocent, amused toddlers beaming out of the patio window were going to be our children.

The Final Furlong

We went into battle for these children against other couples and we won. The twins would be ours. Our hearts have never been so full, the joy spilling over.

Unofficially, Jojo had done some detective work once she had been officially informed that we would be adopting the twins. She found me on Facebook, we have been chatting ever since, in her first message to me she shared new firsts for the twins and sent a couple more recent photographs. Clandestine communication! I was thrilled to be breaking the rules after so long of toeing the line. I was not sorry, just living in my warm and fuzzy feelings and feeding my need for knowledge.

Our introduction day had finally arrived, and Louisa was driving us to meet the twins. I sat in the back of the car and left Henri and Louisa to chat in the background as I receded into my own space. I watched as the meandering countryside fell away to larger more purposeful main roads as we headed somewhere new. Containing myself in the back seat was hard. Just one more hour, one more hour after years of waiting. I expected the rampant anxiety monkey to be causing havoc, but it was quiet today, maybe even the monkey knew this day was important to stay in the moment, to savour the first time. I wasn't giving birth today, but it was as close as I was going to get to it. A momentous occasion and expectations swung from being high to reigning that vibration into a more manageable level. I wanted to be consumed with them, their smell, their sounds, how they felt in my lap. I was impatient, the roads were long, and Louisa was a slow, cautious driver.

Eventually, we turned off the main road and went down a series of roads leading to a quiet, leafy residential area; trees lined the pavements and houses were tucked securely behind neatly trimmed bushes and wooden gates. Louisa's car slowed and pulled up to the curb in front of a sand-coloured house with a decently sized driveway with a family car parked on it. There's not much else to see from my misty car window. The others climbed out and I just sat there, unable to move, suddenly frozen with fear. What if they don't like me? What if I don't like them? What if I can't do this? What if I end up being a terrible mother? So many what-ifs flying around my head. Henri opened my door. "Ready?" He took my hand and pulled me out of my spiral and onto the driveway.

Louisa rang the doorbell, and we stood back behind her, waiting, almost hiding a little. This is it. A dog barked; a child shrieked. "Coming!" Jojo yelled.

She opened the door with a huge smile, "Welcome, oh it's so, so good to meet you." She winked at me. "Come in, come in. Don't worry about shoes; we are going through a refit, and you know twin toddlers and teens make a lot of mess. It's just how it is! Pop your coats on the stairs and come in."

I hung back a bit, suddenly feeling a shyness I've not felt since I was a child, although that was quickly replaced with nervous laughter as my crotch was filled with the snout of a big drooling French Mastiff. "Oh Wilma, get away." Jojo pulled her away and we bundled into the living room where two pairs of curious eyes met us. The little girl was standing up, holding onto the sofa and the boy rolled around giggling on the floor. "Jojo!" The girl demanded Jojo's attention and stuck her hand in the air to make her point. Jojo picked her up and walked her over to Henri. Henri and the little girl locked eyes and she reached for him. He took her gently into his arms and sat down with her on his lap. She grinned at him and then toppled into his chest, where she stayed for a while. She looked like she had found something special. The little boy started to play with his toy cars, "Brum brum. Beep beep," so I sat myself down next to Henri to watch him. I had completely lost the ability to speak. Sensing this, Louisa started a conversation with Jojo about how they were doing.

"Right, let's get some hot drinks. Tea? Coffee?" Jojo walked out of sight with Louisa into the kitchen. She popped her head back in, "I'll just grab these and then I'll be back then we can chat about the twins' history."

We were left alone. Henri was so engrossed talking to the little girl he didn't even notice that we had been left alone. He pulled out his phone. "I've got someone very important to show you. He is going to be your big furry brother." He pulled up a photo of Digby. "This is your dog Digby. Can you say Digby?"

"Bigby!" She shrieked with delight and grabbed the phone and kissed his screen giggling as she did so! Oh, my heart.

Jojo had told them that we were Mama and Dadda right from when she found out we were to be their parents. She had referred to us always with those names so when the little boy offered me a car to play with, "Mmmmmammmm ta!" Jojo was back with cups of milky coffee in time to hear him, she praised him, "Yes this is mama, well done!" The grin on my face was so wide it threatened to slide off the edges. I have never felt such a surge of love towards anything the way I did in that moment.

Mama.

That afternoon we learnt a lot more about the twins' history and the trauma it had brought with it. They had a road of recovery ahead of them and we would be their safe place, their guide, their go-to, their parents.

Both Henri and I had a go at changing nappies, feeding them, reading them books, and playing with them. When we went to leave, they started to cry. Jojo reassured us, "It's ok they've missed their nap; they are tired and hungry. So, close your ears Louisa, if you want to come down for an afternoon before Christmas you are very welcome."

"Jojo don't encourage them; oh I am not listening! I'll see you two at the car." She grinned and made for the door.

I smile. "I would like to. Sorry Louisa, you didn't hear that."

"Just don't tell me, right let's get going. Thanks Jojo!"

We did sneak down and see the twins before Christmas, we spent a blissful afternoon with Jojo and playing with the twins. Christmas was all around us, and I finally understood why parents always say the season is really all about the children. The joy in their faces as they watch the lights twinkle on the tree, curiously touching the forbidden shiny baubles when they think no one is watching, reading books, and learning about Father Christmas and his elves, greedily scoffing down chocolate coins as treats. We got to bathe them this time and help put them down for a nap. We came home feeling a little drunk in love with these two funny, mischievous toddlers.

Our very last hurdle to jump over was a trip back to the Panel room for approval from the Matching Panel to adopt them. It was January and a bleak day outside, but nothing could deter us from feeling upbeat and hopeful. Not today. Marjory was back in the room and was delighted to see us back so soon. She watched as the twins reached for us when they came into the room. The little boy delighted by the amount of attention he was getting broke into his rendition of Baa Baa Black Sheep. Everyone clapped and the twins shrieked in delight. Jojo submitted her report approving our adoption of her twin wards from her point of view. The Panel unanimously agreed we would officially be able to adopt the twins and ordered that the handover period be organised immediately. They also approved a name change which was good, as we had already chosen new names and Jojo had already started calling them by these new names from when we saw them all pre-Christmas.

To celebrate we asked Jojo if we could all go for supper in the local town, and she thought this would be a super idea. We all bundled into a brightly lit noodle bar from outside in the cold and dark late afternoon. We ordered and the twins threw noodles everywhere, covering every inch of their faces with sauce. Coming back from the toilet, I looked over towards them all, this is my family. My new family. My heart burst open.

The two-week handover happened in January, not unlike the two-week wait to see if I was pregnant after IVF, it was long and emotional. All we wanted was to scoop them up and bring them home. The first week consisted of us travelling to them daily to get immersed in their routine. We needed to be there when they woke up and when they went to bed, they needed to know we were their normal. We fed them, changed nappies, played, bathed them, dealt with tantrums, read to them, hugged them, rocked them to sleep in our laps, talked to them about us and our lives (of course they didn't understand), watched Peppa Pig with them and fed them bottles of warm milk. The days were full.

Our first time taking them out started by needing help to fit car seats, it took three of us thirty minutes before giving up and calling for the help of Jojo's teenage son. We wrapped them up and strapped them in. I started the engine, looked behind me to check they were OK and drove off towards the park. "I feel a huge responsibility driving our precious cargo. Every time I look in my rear-view mirror, I see two pairs of beautiful eye staring back at me, trusting us to do the right thing by them."

"Yup it's mental. These are our children. Mama and Daddy. Scary. I wonder if all new parents feel this way. You know you are doing twenty-five in a forty, don't you?" I grin at him.

We pushed them on the swings and when the light started to fail, we took them to soft play. We had never been inside a soft play before. Bold, bright primary colours screamed at us in forms of foam shapes, little balls in a pit, shiny slides, and netting. It was loud. Children running everywhere, laughing, shouting, crying, tantrumming and sleeping. Sleeping amongst this chaos, imagine that! The twins were small toddlers, so I think people assumed we knew what we were doing, so asking a thousand questions to the teenage receptionists drew some strange glances. When we ordered the twins two plates of fish fingers, chips, and baked beans we were asked what size. "Yeah, you know normal size." The plates of hot food arrived on big plates, and we popped them in front of the twins. The plates were bigger than their heads. Buddie, our boy twin poured his beans over his head then smeared it down his face and then laughed hysterically. Dolly, our little girl laughed as she chewed on a chip before spitting it out in favour of a fish finger. They ate barely anything, and we had learnt our first parenting lesson.

Week two was Jojo's turn to drive the twins to us to get them familiar with their new home and meet Digby. Digby took to them straight away, his belly providing an important cushion to take naps on. Slowly Jojo left us alone with them in our home for longer and longer, then came the sleepover day. Jojo arrived not just with the twins but with some of their toys she had bought them and a bag of clothes each. Dolly was not in the best mood that day and was displaying quite clingy behaviour with Jojo. Louisa turned up too and we all sat about over tea and an alarming amount of coloured plastic toys discussing the next steps. Jojo left the room for the bathroom and Dolly started to cry which turned into screaming with huge, fat tears rolling down her face. Henri picked her up which soothed her a little. I stepped out to talk to Jojo. "What do you think Jojo, I can see you are worried."

"Well, the thing with Dolly is that she is very attached to me. She will be fine, but it will take her some time to settle. I am not worried about leaving her because today is about you and Henri and the family coming together. She is in more than capable hands with you and Henri, I truly believe that. I guess I am just sad I suppose that today she is having an off day."

"Louisa thinks that we should not do the sleepover today but tomorrow instead."

"I think we should do it today. I'll come back and check in tomorrow with the remainder of their things. It will all be OK."

We chatted some more, Dolly calmed down and started playing again. Jojo got up signalling to me to follow her. She whispered, "OK I am off. You guys have got this. Call me if you need me, I am going to make a quick exit." With that she picked up her bag, swung it on her shoulder, bent down to the twins. "Jojo says be good, OK? See you tomorrow," and then she was gone. Louisa had left before her; we were left alone.

The five of us were alone for the first time.

We laughed. No one but us. The twins looked at us and laughed too. We scooped them up and sank into the sofa to watch some kids' TV. Digby, exhausted from his day being a new plaything retreated to the quiet of the hallway and his bed.

....

Dolly and Buddie were seventeen months old when they came home to live with us on the 28th January 2016. They settled in with Digby at their side wherever they went, his new bed dragged by him to sleep just inside their bedroom threshold, keeping them safe. They had to climb over him when they woke from naps. He was an old dog now, but he loved them and allowed them to climb all over him, pull his fur and play with his ears. When they fell, he nudged them up encouraging them to try again. As he was going deaf, he didn't really mind the new continuous shrieking, crying and chatter that had taken over from just our gentle voices. He especially loved it when they fell asleep on his belly. Digby, like us, was smitten.

Postscript

We are now in 2025 and the twins are ten years old, and full of life and character. Settling in with us took a good year and a half and we are still working through some of the trauma they came with. As twins they are the ying and yang of each other. One has blue eyes, the other brown, one loves marmite the other hates it! One is left-handed and very outgoing and the other is right-handed and an observer, the quiet one. It is true to say they turned our lives upside down, but we don't care, they are our children and our family, and we love them as hard as any parent loves their children.

We all cried a lot a few years ago when we lost Digby in that February. He was sixteen years old and the best furry big brother they could have ever had. We miss him enormously and I often find biscuits, toys and little notes left in his old sleeping spot gifted from the twins, each time I find them my heart breaks a little but then I remember the sunshine he brought them and us, and I will be forever grateful to him, my boy, my wonderful furry boy.

Acknowledgement

Huge thank you to my husband, Henri. You believe in me without question, and I am so grateful to you. Without you none of this would have been possible, the story itself or the space to write it. My constant, my love.

Our twins, you are now ten and about to go to secondary school, how has time warped so fast that you are now this grown up! It's been a wild ride, and we have loved all of it, even the tough times as you showed us what it looks like to have courage and be brave enough to keep moving forward. You are both incredible humans and we are privileged to have you in our lives.

A special thank you to Jo Russell, for so many reasons but largely for being the best foster mama we could have hoped for with the twins, and for providing me with all the information I needed for this book to be as factual as possible with the twin's early life. Combined with police and social worker reports we got the full picture. Not only that, your friendship to me has been such a support. We love you so much Jojo.

Huge thank you to our family and friends for your unwavering support. You have all been such fantastic humans. Special mention to my sister Angela, Annette our wonderful beam of light, Louise W for her honestly and keeping it real, Emma for her broad shoulders and lifts and Tot and Vic C who plied me with plenty of tea and sage advice.

Massive thank you to my two wonderful beta readers: Kate and Sadie, your input was so appreciated.

Lastly, to our soul dog, Digby. I used your fur to wipe my tears more times than I care to admit, you were always by my side then you made room for the twins too. You are gone now but never forgotten, the twins still leave you biscuits where you used to sleep. We miss you immeasurably and you will always have a place in our hearts.

www.ingramcontent.com/pod-product-compliance
Lightning Source LLC
Chambersburg PA
CBHW020412080526
44584CB00014B/1299